Diet Against Disease

Also by Alice A. Martin

All About Apples

Also by Frances Tenenbaum

Gardening with Wild Flowers
Nothing Grows for You?
Plants from Nine to Five
Over 55 Is *Not* Illegal

Diet Against Disease

A New Plan for Safe and Healthy Eating

Alice A. Martin
and Frances Tenenbaum

Houghton Mifflin Company
Boston   1980

Library of Congress Cataloging in Publication Data
Martin, Alice A
    Diet Against Disease.

    Includes index.
    1. Nutrition.   2. Diet.   3. Nutritionally
induced diseases.   4. Food.   5. Cookery.
I. Tenenbaum, Frances, joint author.   II. Title.
[DNLM: 1. Nutrition — Popular works.   2. Diet —
Adverse effects — Popular works.   3: Nutrition disorders
— Prevention and control — Popular works.   QU145 M378p]
RA784.M3617   613.2   80-12296
ISBN 0-395-29451-7

Printed in the United States of America
V 10 9 8 7 6 5 4 3 2 1

Acknowledgments

The authors are grateful for the help and guidance of Dr. D. Mark Hegsted, formerly advisor to the Senate Select Committee on Nutrition and now director of the Human Nutrition Center of the United States Department of Agriculture, and of Dr. William E. Connor, professor of medicine at the University of Oregon and director of its Health Sciences Center. The staffs of the libraries of the American Academy of Medicine and Houghton Mifflin Company were most helpful, as were members of the staffs of the Senate Select Committee and the Department of Agriculture. Dr. Michael Jacobson of the Center for Science in the Public Interest and Arlene Bickel of the National Heart and Lung Institute, among many other people, were generous in sharing information with us. The responsibility for the material in this book is, however, ours alone.

Contents

Part III   Recipes and Cooking Procedures   145

Part I

Dietary Factors in Disease

CHAPTER 1

The Dietary Goals

IN BITS AND PIECES over the years, the evidence has been
piling up: something is wrong with the way we eat. An additive here, a sugar substitute there, too much salt, too little
fiber, bacon may cause cancer, and eggs give you a heart attack. Even as we look for the word *polyunsaturated* on the
label, we become saturated with conflicting news bulletins
about food. Meanwhile, as we debate the virtues or dangers
of an individual substance, some say we are missing the
real issue, which is that our whole way of eating may be
hazardous to our health.

Is there really a relationship between the "best" diet in
the world and the epidemic levels of cancer, heart disease,
diabetes, and hypertension that we are seeing today in our
country? If so, what is the connection and what, if anything,
can we do about it?

In the late 1970s, the Senate Select Committee on Nutrition and Human Needs, which previously had been concerned with programs designed to eliminate hunger, began
to investigate a different kind of malnutrition (literally, bad
nutrition), the kind associated with overconsumption. The
committee's action was a response to the growing concern of
consumers, nutritionists, and doctors about the accumulation of scientific data linking diet to the nation's "killer
diseases."

In the very first hearings, patterns linking diet to the exis-
tence of diseases in certain population groups began to

emerge. During the Diet and Cancer hearings, scientific witnesses made the following observations:

• Deaths from colon and breast cancer are uncommon in countries with diets low in animal and dairy fats.
• Groups whose diets are low in fat and at the same time high in dietary fiber have much lower rates of cancers of the colon, rectum, breast, and uterus than comparable groups of Americans who consume more fat and less dietary fiber.
• Japanese who migrate to the United States and change to a Western diet from their traditional Japanese diet (which contains little animal fat and almost no dairy products) dramatically increase their incidence of breast and colon cancer.
• Fat people have a higher risk of developing cancer — particularly cancers of the uterus, breast, and gall bladder — than do people of normal weight.

Dr. Gio Gori, deputy director of the National Cancer Foundation, told the committee that

in the United States the number of cancer cases a year that appear to be related to diet are estimated to be 40 percent of the total incidence for males and about 60 percent of the total incidence for females. The forms of cancer that appear to be dependent on nutrition as shown by epidemiological studies include: stomach, liver, breast, prostate, large intestine, small intestine, and colon. There are other forms of cancer for which evidence is being collected, but as yet, strong evidence is not available.

Dr. Gori concluded, "I want to emphasize we are not saying that there is a direct relationship between diet and cancer. We do have strong clues that dietary factors play a predominant role in the development of these tumors."

Other hearings, different diseases, more testimony, but the same conclusion: diet is related to strokes, heart attacks, cancer, arteriosclerosis, cirrhosis of the liver, and diabetes — six of the ten leading causes of death in America.

As a result of the overwhelming evidence linking diet to

disease, the Senate Select Committee on Nutrition recommended some major changes in the way we eat. What these are, why they are desirable, and specifically how to incorporate them into your own way of eating are the subjects of this book. To understand them, it is first necessary to look briefly at the diet that has got us where we are today — overweight and at risk of disease.

We are a sedentary people compared to Americans who lived before the early 1900s with no cars, no mechanized factories, and no labor-saving devices, yet we consume almost as many calories today as they did then. Though obesity is linked to diabetes, heart disease, and high blood pressure, fifteen million of us are obese to an extent that seriously raises our risk of ill health. And we are getting fatter every day. In 1974, according to a study by the Center for Health Statistics, women under 45 weighed an average of 4.7 pounds more than they did just *twelve* years earlier. The average increase for men under 45 was 3.8 pounds.

Except for the number of calories we consume, our diet has otherwise changed drastically in the past fifty or sixty years, with great and often harmful effects upon our health. Although it is bad enough that we are eating too much for our level of activity, the problem is compounded by the kind of calories we are consuming. Compared with the early 1900s, we are eating one-third more fat, 50 percent more refined sugar, and almost 50 percent less starch. We're eating the same amount of protein, but we're getting much more of it from meat and other fat-rich sources.

By the end of the 1970s, 60 percent of all the calories we consumed each day were in the form of fat and sugar — 20 percent in sugar, which contains no vitamins and minerals, and 40 percent in fat, a relatively poor source of nutrients. We each drank an average of 295 12-ounce cans of soda a year. More than 60 percent of all our food had undergone some form of processing, with consequent loss in nutrients and gain in additives. Not counting sugar and salt, more than 1300 additives had been approved for our food supply. Other things get into it by accident.

While this, briefly, is a description of the diet that has

been implicated in today's epidemic level of certain serious diseases, it is important to understand that there is not a direct cause-and-effect relationship between diet and disease — as there is, for example, between eating lead paint and getting lead poisoning. It is not possible to say that a specific person who eats the average American diet will get cancer. Nor is it possible to say (as some recent books have) that an individual can prevent cancer by changing his or her diet. The evidence of the relationship between diet and disease — and it is overwhelming — is epidemiological: in studies of different population groups, there is a distinct relationship between their diet and their incidence of disease.

Poor diet, therefore, is a risk factor, and risk factors are warning flags. While risk factors cannot tell us about the specific fate of any one person within a population group, they can tell us about the *probability* of an event happening. If your diet resembles that of a group of people with a high incidence of one or more diseases, you increase the probability that you will have that same health problem.

Some risk factors, like age, income, occupation, or the genes we were born with are beyond our control. But diet is one factor that is not, and, as we can see in the chart on the next page, the ability to control this particular risk may be the difference between life and death. Of the ten risk factors associated with heart disease, *seven* are directly related to diet.

Given the indisputable linkage between the average American diet and at least six major diseases, the Senate Select Committee on Nutrition and its scientific advisors drew up a set of guidelines for dietary changes designed to reduce the diet risk factors in disease. Published as the *Dietary Goals for the United States*, the thrust of the recommendations is that we should reduce our intake of sugar, salt, overall fat, saturated fat, red meat, and cholesterol, and increase our consumption of fruits, vegetables, whole grains, and polyunsaturated fats. Although the resulting way of eating would be dramatically different from the average American's

SOME RISK FACTORS ASSOCIATED WITH HEART DISEASE

RISK FACTORS	PHYSIOLOGICAL RESULT	END RESULT
Eating and drinking too much Not exercising enough	} Overweight	}
High total fat consumption High saturated fat consumption Low polyunsaturated: saturated fat ratio High cholesterol consumption	} Elevated blood cholesterol	} Higher risk of heart disease
High salt consumption Overweight	} Elevated blood pressure	
Diabetes Smoking	} Accelerates the atherosclerotic process	}

diet — and is not without its critics — the committee's recommendations coincide almost exactly with the advice of a group of 200 scientists from twenty-three countries. As reported in the *Journal of the American Medical Association* in June 1977, the scientists, who virtually unanimously agreed that there was a relationship between diet and heart disease, suggested the following dietary changes, in order of priority:

Fewer total calories
Less fat
Less saturated fat
Less cholesterol
More polyunsaturated fat
Less sugar
Less salt
More fiber
More starchy foods

In setting the Dietary Goals for the United States, the Senate committee spelled out its recommendations primarily in terms of percentages of caloric intake. Since, quite obviously, it is not possible for the average person to measure the percentages of the various elements that make up the foods in a total daily diet, the committee also made a number of suggestions about how to change our diet to meet the intent of the goals.

The Goals

1. To avoid overweight, consume only as much energy (calories) as expended; if overweight, decrease energy intake and increase energy expenditure. In other words, eat less and exercise more.

2. Increase the consumption of complex carbohydrates and "naturally occurring" sugars from about 28 percent of energy intake to about 48 percent of energy intake. These complex carbohydrates and naturally occurring sugars are the ones found in fruits, vegetables, and whole grains.

3. Reduce the consumption of refined and processed sugars by about 45 percent to account for about 10 percent of total energy intake.

4. Reduce overall fat consumption from approximately 40 percent to about 30 percent of energy intake.

5. Reduce saturated fat consumption to account for about 10 percent of total energy intake; and balance that with polyunsaturated and monounsaturated fats, which should account for about 10 percent of energy intake each.

6. Reduce cholesterol consumption to about 300 milli-grams a day.

7. Limit sodium intake by reducing the intake of salt to about 5 grams a day.

(The diet-disease factors behind these goals are discussed in the chapters that follow.)

How to Change Your Diet to Meet the Goals

1. Increase consumption of fruits and vegetables and whole grains.

2. Decrease consumption of refined and processed sugars and foods high in such sugars.

3. Decrease consumption of foods high in total fat, and partially replace saturated fats, whether obtained from ani-mal or vegetable sources, with polyunsaturated fats.

4. Decrease consumption of animal fat, and choose meats, poultry, and fish that will reduce saturated fat intake.

5. Except for very young children, substitute low-fat and nonfat milk for whole milk, and low-fat dairy products for high-fat dairy products.

6. Decrease consumption of butterfat, eggs, and other high-cholesterol sources. Some consideration should be given to easing the cholesterol goal for premenopausal women, young children, and the elderly in order to obtain the nutritional benefits of eggs in the diet.

7. Decrease consumption of salt and foods high in salt.

(Guidelines for food selection and recipes based on these recommendations appear in Parts II and III.)

• • •

In 1980, the Federal government, in what the *New York Times* called "an historic step," issued a set of dietary guide-lines that "represent the first step toward a national nutri-tion policy that could ultimately reshape the way Americans eat." The guidelines, which appear in the appendix of this book, were issued jointly by the Department of Agriculture and the Department of Health, Education, and Welfare and were endorsed by the surgeon general. Although not specific in terms of the amount of each type of food we should eat, the guidelines are similar to — and, in fact, were clearly derived from — the Dietary Goals.

While the goals are more specifically helpful to individuals who want to take control of their own nutrition, the guidelines are indeed an historic step. For the first time, the federal agencies responsible for food policies, programs, and regulations have come out on the side of consumer and health advocates to agree that we are eating too much fat, too much cholesterol, too much sugar, too much salt — and drinking too much alcohol — and that there is a relationship between this diet and certain serious diseases.

The guidelines will influence the new food-labeling laws, expected to be issued by the time this book is out. They will also, it is expected, lead to an overhaul in meat grading, which now puts a premium on meat with the highest fat content. They are already having an effect on school lunch programs. The Agriculture Department, which supplies food for schools, is now buying ground beef with no more than 22 percent fat, canned meat and poultry with no more than 1 percent salt, and canned fruits packed in light rather than heavy syrup. Moreover, all schools participating in the lunch programs must now ban the sale of candy, sodas, and gum until after the lunch period.

By understanding the relationship of diet to disease and by following the Dietary Goals, we can all take responsibility for our own health, so far as it is affected by the food we eat. We call this protective nutrition. Practicing protective nutrition cannot assure that you will not get a disease, but it can reduce the probability by reducing the known dietary risk. In spite of the high promises of their titles, so-called anticancer diets or save-your-life diets can do no more. Because these diets are geared to preventing one kind of disease, they actually can do less. Protective nutrition is a much broader way of looking at what we eat; it includes the dietary risks in all of the major killer diseases, not just cancer.

Before the publication of *Dietary Goals*, traditional nutritional advice was pretty well expressed in one sentence: "Eat sensibly, selecting foods from the four basic food groups (meat, dairy products, grains, and fruits and vegetables)." Obviously, someone who doesn't eat a lot of highly processed junk food is going to be healthier than the person who consumes quantities of soda, potato chips, and instant soups, but the four-food-group advice is misleading because it does not make distinctions between "good" foods and "bad" foods within the groups. Although the relationship between saturated fats and cholesterol and heart disease has long been known, the typical four-food-group diet does not mention the need to eat fewer eggs, to choose lean meats over fatty ones, or to select skim-milk dairy products over full-fat foods. No restrictions are placed on the amount of salt or sugar in the daily diet.

Beyond the Goals

In restricting itself to the major diet-disease connections, the Select Committee on Nutrition did not concern itself with vitamins and only touched on the additives in highly processed foods (although admitting that these *are* a problem). While vitamin and mineral deficiencies are not a major nutritional concern in this country — contrary to what one might believe from the sales of these supplements — they are a potential hazard for the person whose diet is high in sugar, which has no vitamins and minerals and high in fat, which has relatively few. They are also a problem in a diet heavily based on processed foods, where many nutrients are lost and only a few are replaced. Parents in particular are rightly concerned with the vitamin and mineral content of foods. Safe, nutritious food is our goal, which means that we should know what vitamins and minerals we need and where to find them, and what additives we can and should avoid, and how to select foods that are free of them.

According to recent polls, Americans are newly and seriously concerned about nutrition — a fact that has not escaped the food manufacturers, who have taken to slapping the word *natural* on any product that can stand it, while at the same time cooking up new chemical feasts to feed our other concern for quick, easy convenience foods. If we are honest, we have to admit that most of us want our nutrition and our junk food too.

While it would be patently untrue to say that home-cooked meals are no more trouble than frozen dinners, good foods can be convenient if you are selective and know what you should look for. Wholesome breads are as easily purchased as the cottony kind; some meats and cheeses have much less fat than others; vegetables differ greatly in vitamin and mineral content; even snack foods can be nutritious. The word *instant* on a food product is more often a slogan than a measure of preparation time: a can of soup, made up of food ingredients, costs less than an instant soup made of chemicals and takes exactly the same time to prepare. Sugar and salt are the major hidden ingredients in most processed foods; simply knowing which products are excessively high in these materials and avoiding them is a step in the right direction that costs nothing in convenience and saves dollars and cents. (So-called convenience foods are invariably more expensive than the ingredients warrant.)

Since the Dietary Goals dictate a fairly drastic change in eating habits, it is not reasonable to expect that you will make these changes easily and completely. But a goal is a goal — something to aim for — and protective nutrition is not an all-or-nothing matter. To whatever degree you change your diet in accordance with the goals, you will reduce the diet-related risk to health. These risks are great but, unlike many of the factors that lead to disease, the *dietary* risks are ones over which we can exercise our own control.

Are the Dietary Goals the perfect answer? According to Dr. D. Mark Hegsted, consultant to the Senate Select Committee and now head of the newly created Human Nutrition Center in the Department of Agriculture:

Many people will say we have not proven our point; we have not demonstrated that the dietary modifications we recommend will yield the dividends expected. We would point out to those people that the diet we eat today was not planned or developed for any purpose. It is a happenstance related to our affluence, the productivity of our farmers, and the activities of our food industry. The risks associated with eating this diet are demonstrably large. The question to be asked, therefore, is not why we should change our diet, but why not? What are the risks associated with eating less meat, less fat, less saturated fat, less cholesterol, less sugar, less salt, and more fruits, vegetables, unsaturated fat, and cereal products — especially whole grain cereals? There are none that can be identified and important benefits can be expected.

CHAPTER 2

Fat

THE EXCESSIVELY HIGH fat intake of the average American, 42 percent of all our calories, has been linked with coronary heart disease and breast and colon cancer, two of the most widely occurring malignancies. Indirectly, since it is the prime cause of obesity, fat has been linked to hypertension, cardiovascular diseases, atherosclerosis, gall bladder disease, hernia, diabetes, and liver diseases.

In light of these alarming connections, the Dietary Goals recommend that Americans

1. decrease consumption of foods high in *total fat* and partially replace *saturated* fats, whether obtained from animal or vegetable sources, with *polyunsaturated* fats.

2. decrease consumption of animal fat and choose meats, poultry, and fish that will reduce saturated fat intake.

3. except for very young children, substitute low-fat and nonfat milk for whole milk and low-fat dairy products for high-fat dairy products.

Fats (more technically, fatty acids) are designated as saturated, monounsaturated, and polyunsaturated. By now, most of us know that saturated fat is bad because it increases the amount of cholesterol in the body, that polyunsaturated fat is good because it *lowers* the body's serum cholesterol, and that monounsaturated fat is neutral, neither good nor bad. Though a gross oversimplification, this is a pretty fair estimate of the role of fat as a risk factor in our diet. It does not, however, include the relationship between *total* fat intake and disease.

Saturated fat, which has the ability to raise plasma cholesterol, a factor in coronary heart disease, is not necessary to human bodily functions. Yet this particular kind of fat currently accounts for 16 percent of our total caloric intake. It is derived primarily from animal sources and is usually, though not always, solid at room temperature.

Monounsaturated fat neither raises nor lowers cholesterol. It is found mostly in plant products, though there are a few animal sources as well. Foods high in monounsaturated fat include lard, some vegetable oils, and some vegetable oil products, particularly the less expensive margarines.

Polyunsaturated fat, the only fat essential to the human diet, contains linoleic acid, which cannot be manufactured by the body and must be taken in as food. Linoleic acid is necessary to maintain cell membrane structure and promote blood clotting time.

Exactly how much fat is needed in our diet, beyond a small amount of linoleic acid, is not known. Although we eat an average of 42 percent of our total calories in the form of fat, during World War II Japanese soldiers lived and functioned on a diet in which, incredibly, only 3 percent of their total calories came from fat. European wartime deprivations, which drastically lowered fat consumption among civilian populations, lowered coronary heart disease rates as well.

In recommending that we decrease our total consumption of fat to 30 percent of our caloric intake — to be divided equally among saturated, monounsaturated, and polyunsaturated fats — the Dietary Goals suggest a very moderate reduction. Using similar recommendations, the Swedish government set an ideal limit of between 25 and 30 percent. However modest the suggested fat reduction is, it will require some important changes in the kind of foods we buy and the way that we prepare them.

First of all, it is important to stress that we need to reduce all fat. Although polyunsaturated fat is capable of lowering serum cholesterol (but only half as effectively as saturated fat elevates it) and is therefore of value in the prevention of heart disease, *all* fat, including polyunsaturated fat, is implicated in obesity and the incidence of breast and colon cancer.

Since we eat most of our fat in the form of meat and dairy products, and since these animal fats are saturated, decreasing fat consumption along the following guidelines will help reduce both total fat and saturated fat.

1. Reduce the amount of meat you eat and select meat, poultry, and fish that are low in fat.

2. Substitute vegetables high in protein — dried peas and beans, grains — for some meat protein.

3. Trim away visible fat from meat, poultry, and fish.

4. Use less fat in cooking and make sure to use polyunsaturated fat.

5. Be aware of the hidden fat in such foods as ice cream, hamburgers, cheese, potato chips, bakery products, mayonnaise, and highly processed foods.

Using the following list, try to select foods that have 30 percent or less of their calories in fat.

Percentage of calories from fat in foods

Over 50 percent from fat

Cream cheese
Frankfurters
Peanuts and peanut butter
Pork lunch meats
Most cheese and cheese spreads
Tongue
Eggs
Regular ground beef
Salmon and tuna fish (packed in oil)
Pork (loin and butt)
Granola

Between 40 percent and 50 percent from fat

Roast chicken, including skin
Beef (porterhouse, T-bone, round rump, lean ground, and
   kidney)
Pork (fresh and cured ham and shoulder)
Lamb (shoulder and rib)
Whole milk
Ice cream

Between 30 percent and 40 percent from fat

Beef (sirloin and flank)
Turkey (dark meat, flesh and skin)
Lamb (loin and leg)

Between 20 percent and 30 percent from fat

Beef (heel of round)
Liver *
Fish (bass and salmon)
Chicken (light meat, roasted or broiled, no skin)

Under 20 percent from fat

Fish (haddock, cod, tuna in water, halibut, sole, and oth-
   ers)
Most shellfish *
Bread
Most peas and beans
Skim-milk cheese
Uncreamed cottage cheese
Skim milk
Most breakfast cereals other than granola-type

(This list was adapted from Ruth Frames and Zak Sabry,
Nutriscore, Methuen/Two Continents Publications, New
York, 1976.)

* Low in fat, but high in cholesterol.

When it comes to replacing part of the saturated fat that we normally eat with polyunsaturated fat, the food advertisers are in there pitching. Before swallowing their wares, however, you should realize that not all vegetable oils are unsaturated and not all margarines are the same. In commercial baked goods, the "pure vegetable oil" on the label is probably coconut oil (86 percent saturated) or palm oil (48 percent saturated) since these are the cheapest vegetable oils. Nondairy creamers and whipped cream substitutes contain coconut oil — with more saturated fat than real cream.

As the table below clearly indicates, the best choices in oils, based on their percentages of polyunsaturated fats, are safflower oil, sunflower oil, and corn oil, in that order. Although olive oil, like coconut oil and palm oil, rates low on the polyunsaturated scale, unlike the other two it also is low in saturated fat. Basically, olive oil is a monosaturated fat, and although it won't help lower serum cholesterol, it is an acceptable occasional choice as a salad dressing.

Margarines and vegetable shortenings such as Crisco start out as liquid vegetable oils. However, when the oil is converted to a solid, some of the liquid oil is hydrogenated, a

PERCENTAGE OF FATTY ACIDS IN COOKING
AND SALAD OILS

OIL	TOTAL FAT	SATURATED FAT	MONO-UNSATURATED FAT	POLY-UNSATURATED FAT
Safflower	100*	9	12	74
Sunflower	100	10	21	64
Corn	100	13	25	58
Soybean	100	14	24	57
Cottonseed	100	26	19	51
Sesame	100	15	40	40
Peanut	100	17	47	31
Palm	100	48	38	9
Olive	100	14	72	9
Coconut	100	86	6	2

*Percentages do not add up to 100 because of minor fat constituents. Table adapted from *Fats in Food and Diet*, U.S. Department of Agriculture Bulletin #361.

PERCENTAGE OF FAT IN SHORTENING, MARGARINE, AND BUTTER

FOOD	TOTAL FAT*	SATURATED FAT	MONO-UNSATURATED FAT	POLY-UNSATURATED FAT
Vegetable shortening	100	25	44	26
Margarine (first ingredient on label):				
Safflower (liquid) tub	80	13	16	48
Corn oil (liquid) tub	80	14	30	32
Corn oil (liquid) stick	80	15	36	24
Soybean (hydrogenated) stick	80	15	46	14
Butter	81	50	23	3

*Percentages do not add up to the total fat percentage because of minor fat constituents. Table adapted from *Fats in Food and Diet*, U.S. Department of Agriculture Bulletin #361.

process that in effect saturates the oil. The best choice in margarines is the one that has a highly unsaturated oil as its first ingredient on the label. As a rule, margarines sold in tubs are less solid than margarines sold by the stick and therefore less hydrogenated.

Although margarines generally have far less saturated fat than butter, they also contain artificial flavoring, preservatives, and other additives. (The artificial color is carotene, a natural source of vitamin A, which is also used in butter.) If this makes margarine unacceptable to you, a reasonable compromise is to use butter at the table and a highly polyunsaturated oil for cooking. In both cases, though, remember that it is important to use distinctly smaller quantities if you're trying to get down to 30 percent fat in your diet.

CHAPTER 3

Cholesterol

CHOLESTEROL IS A fat-soluble substance that is synthesized only by animal organisms. We manufacture it in our own bodies and eat it in the form of animal products. In the marketplace, vegetable-oil manufacturers vie with each other in touting their products as containing "no cholesterol." *No* vegetable product contains cholesterol.

Basic to any discussion of cholesterol is an understanding of the distinction between *plasma* (or serum) cholesterol and *dietary* cholesterol.

Plasma cholesterol exists in small amounts in almost all cells and is vital to human functioning. It is carried through the bloodstream by a group of substances known as lipoproteins. The amount of plasma cholesterol, that is, cholesterol in the bloodstream, is accepted as a good indicator of the risk of heart disease. The higher one's level of plasma cholesterol, the higher one's risk of having heart disease. Likewise, it has been shown that the lower one's level of plasma cholesterol, the lower one's risk of this disease.

Dietary cholesterol is the cholesterol we eat. Research indicates that diets that are high in dietary cholesterol and/or saturated fats raise the level of plasma cholesterol. Conversely, a low-cholesterol diet and/or a diet high in polyunsaturated fats tends to lower the total plasma cholesterol.

This research also indicates that lowering the intake of saturated fat has a larger impact on plasma cholesterol than does lowering the intake of dietary cholesterol.

In the United States, according to *Dietary Goals*, many doctors consider a plasma cholesterol range of between 200–300 milligrams to be normal. However, normal is not optimal, nor does it imply any protection from heart disease. In fact, a cholesterol level of 260 milligrams or higher carries with it five times the risk for heart disease as compared to a level of 220 milligrams or less. Only in societies where the level of plasma cholesterol is under 150 or 160 milligrams do we find virtually no deaths from heart disease. Interestingly, babies all over the world have cholesterol levels of about 70–90 milligrams at birth.

Indeed, the process of developing heart disease begins in childhood, as cholesterol deposited in the walls of the arteries begins to form a plaque. As the plaque continues to build up in the arteries, it reduces the flow of blood. This partial or full blockage in the coronary arteries eventually leads to reduced function, causing the severe chest pains of angina pectoris, heart attacks, and death.

The role of plasma and dietary cholesterol in the development of heart disease has probably received more attention than any other nutritional research issue. One of the most significant research concerns has been the investigation of lipoproteins, which are the carriers of cholesterol and other fatty substances in the bloodstream. Two lipoproteins have been found to be of particular interest: LDL, or low-density lipoproteins, and HDL, high-density lipoproteins.

High levels of cholesterol-rich LDL *have been directly correlated with heart disease*, and the level of LDL is *directly related to the consumption of dietary cholesterol and fat*.

HDL not only carries less cholesterol than does LDL; it also appears to be protective with respect to heart disease. In other words, the higher one's HDL level, the lower the risk of having heart disease. On the other hand, the amount of fat in the diet doesn't seem to have any effect on the HDL level, which does seem to be increased by exercise, niacin, and estrogens. More recently, another form of HDL called HDLc has been discovered that seems to act as a cholesterol-*depositing* agent. The predictive value of LDL and HDL is not at present being utilized by physicians. However, since the LD level is related to one's diet and the HDL level is influenced by exercise, the obvious answer for an individual is to exercise more and eat the lower-fat, lower-cholesterol diet recommended by the Dietary Goals.

In addition to dietary factors that affect the level of an individual's plasma cholesterol, there are also metabolic factors. Briefly, there is a mechanism in the liver that controls the synthesis of cholesterol — when cholesterol is not present in the diet, the body can make all that it needs. Conversely, when dietary cholesterol is available, the body's own production will be inhibited. However, researchers have found that this control mechanism cannot completely compensate for the amount of cholesterol in the diet, and they have concluded that the best way to control the level of plasma cholesterol is through diet modification.

In the Dietary Goals, this modification covers both intake of fat (as discussed in the previous chapter) and a 300-milligram-per-day limit on dietary cholesterol.

The table on page 24 gives the cholesterol content of common measures of selected foods.

Looking at this list, it becomes clear that there are relatively few foods to be completely avoided. Brains and kidneys are not the most tempting of delicacies for most Americans in any event. Although liver is a superior source of iron, not many of us eat it every day. The egg is another story.

In regard to the cholesterol issue, the Select Committee on Nutrition received "countless" questions, comments, and suggestions. In general, they focused on two basic areas:

1. Does the cholesterol recommendation apply to the general population or only to people at high risk of heart disease?
2. What does this mean for egg consumption, which is the single largest source of cholesterol in the American diet?

In its preface to the second edition of *Dietary Goals for the United States*, published in 1977, the Senate Select Committee responded to these issues:

The 300 mg per day recommendation does not mean eliminating egg consumption. Nor does it imply that one should replace eggs with one of the highly processed egg-substitutes or imitation egg products.

Eggs are an excellent, inexpensive source of protein, vitamins and minerals. The 250 mg of cholesterol in an average egg, as well as the bulk of the calories, is contained in the yolk. As a result, some researchers advocate using in one's diet only egg whites . . .

Finally, one should view cholesterol as only one component of a total diet. We recommend a general level of cholesterol consumption, and leave the ultimate source of that dietary component up to the consumer. Since eggs are only one source of dietary cholesterol, a specific recommendation as to the number of eggs necessary to meet the goal is inappropriate.

Keeping in mind that the risk of heart disease is significantly lower among women until they reach menopause, and that young children and the elderly need particularly good sources of high quality protein, vitamins and minerals, it may be advisable for persons in these groups to include more eggs in their diet — even to the point of easing the cholesterol recommendation in order to increase egg consumption.

It is not possible to say exactly how much to ease the recommendation since no scientific panels have specifically set cholesterol intake levels for population sub-groups. In suggesting that the cholesterol might be eased for young children, pre-menopausal women and the elderly in order to obtain the nutritional benefits of additional eggs, the Select Committee does remain concerned as to what happens when the period of reduced risk is over and possible cumulative effects from the diet take place.

In summary, the Select Committee understands that there is still controversy surrounding the exact relationship of dietary cholesterol to heart disease, and that we must aggressively continue research in order to bring resolution to the current dispute. However, over the last 25 years, there has been a steady and mounting accumulation of basic research and epidemiological evidence which indicates that a high plasma cholesterol level is a major risk factor in heart disease and that dietary cholesterol is one of a number of factors which affects plasma cholesterol. As one result, ten national and international panels have recommended the restriction of dietary cholesterol for the general population.

This past year, Dr. Robert Levy, Director, National Heart, Lung and Blood Institute, National Institutes of Health, announced that recent surveys suggest that the average American's plasma cholesterol level has dropped five to ten percent since the early 1960's, which may have contributed to the sharp decline in deaths from heart and blood vessel diseases over the last several years.

As public policymakers, the members of the Select Committee cannot ignore the known findings which indicate the high probability that cholesterol intake contributes to the development of cardiovascular disease. The Select Committee cannot ignore the fact that 850,000 Americans die each year from heart and blood vessel disease, that 50 percent of all deaths are related to cardiovascular

CHOLESTEROL CONTENT OF COMMON MEASURES OF SELECTED FOODS

FOOD	AMOUNT	CHOLESTEROL (MG)
Skim milk, fluid or reconstituted dry	1 cup	5
Uncreamed cottage cheese	½ cup	7
Light cream	1 ounce	20
Creamed cottage cheese	½ cup	26
Regular ice cream (10 percent fat)	½ cup	27
Cheddar cheese	1 ounce	28
Whole milk	1 cup	34
Butter	1 tablespoon	35
Oysters, salmon	3 ounces, cooked	40
Clams, halibut, tuna	3 ounces, cooked	55
Light meat chicken, turkey	3 ounces, cooked	67
Beef, pork, lobster, dark meat chicken and turkey	3 ounces, cooked	75
Lamb, veal, crab	3 ounces, cooked	85
Shrimp	3 ounces, cooked	130
Beef heart	3 ounces, cooked	230
Egg	1 yolk or 1 egg	250
Liver	3 ounces, cooked	370
Kidney	3 ounces, cooked	680
Brains	3 ounces, raw	more than 1700

Adapted from *Fats in Food and Diet*, U.S. Department of Agriculture Bulletin #361.

illness, which, either directly or indirectly, costs the Nation over $50 billion annually. Heart disease is America's number one killer.

It therefore seems that the only prudent course of action to take in the best interest of the health of the Nation is to recommend that cholesterol consumption be reduced to about 300 mg a day.

CHAPTER 4

Protein

WHEN THE FIRST EDITION of *Dietary Goals* was published, the Senate Select Committee on Nutrition was both congratulated and condemned, depending on the point of view of the respondents, for recommending a "semi-vegetarian" diet. At issue were the goals on reducing overall fat and, specifically, saturated fat, which the committee suggested we could achieve "by reducing consumption of meat and increasing consumption of fish." Needless to say, the meat industry was less than happy with this recommendation.

In the second edition of *Dietary Goals*, in reaction to industry protests, the committee changed its advice from "decrease consumption of meat" to "decrease consumption of animal fat, and choose meats, poultry and fish which will reduce saturated fat intake."

As a political gesture, this change appears to soften the stand on meat; in practice, it doesn't really affect it. While the committee was careful to point out that it "did not indicate a preference for vegetable over animal protein," neither did it recommend a change in the present 12 percent total protein in the diet. Therefore, if you follow the recommendations to increase the consumption of whole grains, fruits, and vegetables, and to reduce saturated fat — while maintaining the same level of protein intake — an alteration in the ratio of animal to vegetable protein inevitably will occur.

Also, while it is politic to suggest that we select meats,

poultry, and fish that are lower in saturated fat, in practice this too means less meat. In steak, the calories are about equally divided between protein and fat. In chicken or fish, however, protein provides about 75 percent of the calories, fat 25 percent or less. (Skim milk, with virtually no fat at all, is 40 percent protein in terms of calories.)

Although the committee did not believe that there is sufficient evidence to recommend a reduction in overall protein intake, it did make some surprising observations.

The first is that the average American eats about twice as much protein as the Food and Nutrition Board of the National Academy of Sciences has set as the Recommended Dietary Allowance (RDA) for most healthy people. *There is no known nutritional need for the amount of protein we eat.*

Second, while our actual protein intake has remained at 12 percent overall since 1909, the ratio of animal protein to vegetable protein has doubled. In 1909, we got 6 percent of our total calories from vegetable protein and 6 percent from animal protein. Today, we get less than 4 percent from vegetables and more than 8 percent from animal foods.

Although heart disease is epidemic in this and other Western countries, it is virtually unknown among population groups whose diets are based on complex carbohydrates and are low in meat and cholesterol. The one population exception is the Eskimo, about whom more later.

A diet that contains twice the RDA for protein can be harmful in other ways too. Too much protein lowers the body's ability to absorb calcium. Meat contains phosphorus, and in overly large amounts, phosphorus can also create a calcium deficiency. In research on rats, in which the animals were fed an amount of protein comparable to twice the RDA for humans (or just about what the average American eats), the rats showed signs of a disorder similar to osteoporosis, the bone disease of older people. Too much protein may also cause a deficiency in vitamin B_6.

The connection between protein and vitamin B_6 is the subject of an interesting new theory on the role of a high-meat diet in the incidence of heart attacks. As opposed to the cholesterol theory, where the villain is presumed to be the saturated fat in meats that acts to elevate plasma cholesterol, this theory holds that it may actually be the *protein* in meat that is the dietary risk for heart disease. This theory, as we will see, would also account for the low incidence of heart attacks among meat-eating Eskimos, because they eat their meat raw.

According to the protein-B_6 theory, whose principal proponent is Dr. Kilmer McCully, a pathologist at the Harvard Medical School, the relationship between methionine, one of the amino acids in protein, and vitamin B_6 is responsible for the presence or absence of atherosclerosis. When there is a deficiency of B_6, methionine produces a toxic substance known as homocysteine, which builds up in the blood. This substance, which, unlike cholesterol, is not normally found in human blood, has been found in significant quantities in the blood of people with heart disease.

Some other evidence bolsters this theory:

• People with heart disease have much lower than normal levels of vitamin B_6.
• The production of the toxic homocysteine can be induced in the body by a diet low in vitamin B_6.
• Oral contraceptives are known to create a vitamin B_6 deficiency. Women who have taken the Pill for as short a time as five years have ten times the normal death rate from heart attacks.

On the other hand, in diets where the ratio of B_6 to the amino acid methionine is high, there is no build-up of homocysteine in the blood, since the vitamin quickly converts it to a harmless substance. The ratio of B_6 to methionine is favorable in fruits and vegetables — which brings us back to the fact that population groups whose dietary intake is based on complex carbohydrates have very few deaths from heart disease. And back to the meat-eating Eskimos.

However, now we can see a difference. Although vitamin B_6 is present in many foods including meat, about half of it is lost in cooking. (In canning, about two-thirds of the vitamin is lost. As much as 90 percent is removed when whole wheat flour is processed into white flour, and B_6 is not one of the vitamins replaced in enriched flour.) So in spite of all the raw meat they eat, the Eskimos might well have an adequate B_6-methionine ratio in their diet, while the diet of the average meat-eating American could easily be deficient.

Whether or not this theory of heart disease ever replaces the plasma cholesterol theory, it gives us an additional reason to limit the amount of meat protein we eat. Since too much protein, as mentioned before, can also create a vitamin B_6 deficiency, it also underlines the need to eat unprocessed foods and vitamin B_6-rich complex carbohydrates.

Considering that we eat double the RDA of protein, and especially considering the demonstrated role of saturated fat in breast and colon cancer as well as heart disease, it would certainly be prudent to cut down on meat, our primary source of saturated fat. Eat chicken and turkey, but remove the skin; lean meats, but cut off all visible fat; and fish. Although shellfish is fine on the fat score, it is high in cholesterol. Organ meats like liver are extremely nutritious but also high in cholesterol. Avoid fatty meats like bacon, frankfurters, sausage, and luncheon meats. If you read Chapter 10 on additives, you will find another compelling reason to drop these foods from the menu.

For the health of your budget as well as your body, it makes sense to replace some meat protein with protein from vegetable sources — dried beans, grains, nuts, and seeds, especially. Except for soybeans, vegetable proteins are incomplete — they lack certain essential amino acids. Most of the protein we consume can be classified as complete or partially complete, depending on its composition. A complete protein can maintain body tissues and sustain normal growth. Eggs, milk, fish, chicken, and meat are examples of complete-protein foods. Wheat germ, dried yeast, and soy products approach these animal products in completeness. Other vegetable proteins — grains and dried legumes — are examples of incomplete-protein foods.

These partially complete proteins will maintain life but cannot support growth. However, when a food lacking in one of the eight essential amino acids is combined with another that compensates for that lack, the body benefits as if a complete protein were consumed. No one who eats some meat or dairy products will suffer a protein deficiency by eating a wide range of chiefly vegetable proteins. Vegan vegetarians, however, will do well to read *Diet for a Small Planet* by Frances Moore Lappe for an excellent explanation of how to combine vegetables to make complete proteins.

Finally, meat is an excellent source of many vitamins and minerals, including some, like iron, that are not otherwise plentiful in our diets. Mild iron deficiency anemia is a not uncommon nutritional disorder, especially among teenagers and premenopausal and pregnant women. On balance, it is better to get one's complement of nutrients such as iron from many sources, including supplements if necessary, than to risk the health hazards associated with a meat-intensive diet.

Protein, as we've always been told, contains the basic building blocks of life. We need protein and we need it every day. But we don't need as much as we eat, on the average, and we don't need it all in the form of meat.

CHAPTER 5

Starch

OF ALL THE DIETARY GOALS, most surprising may be the goal that urges, "Increase the consumption of complex carbohydrates and 'naturally occurring' sugars from about 28 percent of energy intake to about 48 percent of energy intake."

In plain English, we are being told to get almost half of our total calories from starchy foods. To a diet-conscious, although not always conscientiously dieting, people, the idea that we will reduce our risks of disease (including the risk that comes from being overweight) by eating more starch requires some explanation.

The first has to do with the sources of "naturally occurring" sugars and complex carbohydrates. Naturally occurring sugars are simple sugars, like the fructose that sweetens fruit. They occur in high-nutrient foods. Double sugars like sucrose (or table sugar) do break down into simple sugars in the body — but there the similarity ends. Unlike fruit or other sources of naturally occurring sugars, sucrose is a pure carbohydrate that not only contains no nutrients, it steals nutrients from the body to complete its metabolism. (Read about sugar in Chapter 6.)

Carbohydrates are one of the three basic organic compounds in foods. The other two are fat and protein.

Plant foods — grains, fruits, and vegetables — in their *unrefined, unprocessed* state, are an important source of complex carbohydrates, vitamins, minerals, even protein. They are the *only* source of the dietary fiber that assists in the digestion of other foods.

If the Dietary Goal for complex carbohydrates merely told us to increase consumption of these foods, without diminishing our intake of other basic foods, the result indeed would be obesity. However, at the same time that we are advised to eat more starch, we are also enjoined to eat less fat and less sugar. At the present time, these two foods make up 60 percent of our total caloric intake.

As for starch being a "fattening" food, the facts belie this misconception. Complex carbohydrates provide exactly the same amount of calories as protein and sugar — 6 calories per gram. (Fat provides 9 calories per gram.) In addition, when it comes to weight control, the high water content and bulk found in fruits, vegetables, and grains can bring a longer lasting satisfaction of appetite than foods with concentrated calories. Clearly, six chocolate kisses (about 160 calories) are not going to be nearly as filling as two slices of whole wheat bread, for the same number of calories.

Since sugar offers no nutrients and fat relatively few for the amount of calories, and since complex carbohydrates are very high in vitamins and minerals, a diet based more heavily on starch is inevitably going to be a more nutritious one. And complex carbohydrates don't carry the disease risks that fat and sugar do. Population studies repeatedly show that people who consume a diet based on complex carbohydrates have low incidences of heart disease and cancer.

Throughout history, complex carbohydrates have been the chief source of energy for the human race. Not until about 1910, in this country, did the emphasis switch from starchy foods to fats as the major energy source. Unfortunately, at the same time that we have come to eat less starch, we have learned to eat it in a nutritionally degraded way. In the process of refining flour, in particular, much of the natural food value in grain is milled out — the bran layer with its fiber and the germ, the primary source of nutrients. What is left is practically pure starch. When flours are enriched, a few nutrients are replaced. Many are not.

With increased use of canned and frozen vegetables, a decline in the use of whole grain products, and a shift away from potatoes and dried legumes, our intake of nutrients has been affected in a measurable way. Specifically, according to a Department of Agriculture report in 1972, our diets are providing considerably less vitamin A, vitamin B_6, thiamine, and magnesium. (A more recent concern is the lack of fiber in our food, which is discussed in Chapter 9.)

Moreover, things are getting worse. Between 1947 and 1976, the average yearly consumption of complex carbohydrate foods changed to the following degree:

Flour and cereal (grain) products — down 31 pounds

Fruits, other than citrus — down 30 pounds

Potatoes — down 21 pounds

Vegetables, other than dark green and deep yellow — down 12 pounds

Dark green and deep yellow vegetables — down 0.3 of a pound

Citrus fruits, including frozen orange juice — up 10.5 pounds

It will take some doing to turn back the clock on complex carbohydrates (we show how in Parts II and III of this book), but if you need an added incentive besides the prospect of better health, there is always your pocketbook. These are our most economical foods.

CHAPTER 6

Sugar

EVERY DAY OF THE YEAR, the average American man, woman, and child eats one-third of a pound — two-thirds of a cup — of sugar. This includes only the sugar that is added to food, not the naturally occurring sugars in fruit, vegetables, and milk. Refined and processed sugars account for 18 percent or almost one-fifth of all the calories we eat each day.

The Dietary Goal for sugar recommends that we decrease consumption by 45 percent, to bring it down to 10 percent of our total calorie intake.

How bad is sugar, and why? Although some antisugar advocates hold it responsible for most of mankind's ailments, there is no clear scientific evidence that sugar is directly related to any life-threatening disease. It is, however, clearly related to obesity, which in turn is a risk factor in heart disease, high blood pressure, and diabetes. And whether or not it is true that sugar causes hyperactivity in children as some claim, it definitely causes cavities, gum disease, and subsequent loss of teeth. According to one government survey, 98 percent of all American children have cavities, and by age 55 half the population has no teeth at all.

In terms of general nutrition and health, perhaps the most serious problem with eating one-fifth of our calories in the form of sugar is that these are "empty" calories. Refined sugar contains no vitamins, no minerals, no protein, no fat — only pure carbohydrates. Almost all other foods contain some combination of essential nutrients; sugar has only calories. If 20 percent of your calories come from sugar, the remaining 80 percent must supply 100 percent of your nutrients. And there's the rub. If you consume a balanced diet as well as large amounts of sugar, you are likely to be overweight. If you cut down on calories but still eat a lot of sugar, you'll be malnourished because there aren't enough calories of real food to supply your body's daily requirements for nutrients. If your high-sugar diet also happens to be high in fat, which is another relatively poor source of nutrients for the amount of calories, the obesity-malnutrition factor is compounded.

But that isn't the end of the problem. Ironically, at the same time that sugar replaces nutritious food, it increases the need for certain nutrients; specifically, the B vitamin thiamine and the trace mineral chromium. Considering the amount of sugar we eat, it should come as no surprise that the average American diet is marginally deficient in thiamin and that some groups, particularly pregnant women and older people, are also deficient in chromium.

A 20-percent-sugar-calorie diet is generally most harmful to growing children, people on diets, and the elderly. Since we require fewer calories as we age, the diet of an older person, if it is heavily based on bakery goods and convenience foods, will be even more disproportionally high in sugar.

The conviction of some dieters that a piece of candy eaten before meals will reduce their appetites is quite simply fallacious. Sugar is so rapidly absorbed in the body that it does not create a feeling of fullness.

Another sugar myth has to do with eating a candy bar for quick energy. This does work for a short time, but the quickly attained high level of blood sugar drops just as quickly, and even further, leaving behind that extreme letdown or shaky feeling described as the sugar blues. Eating protein and the complex carbohydrates, which are digested more slowly, is the way to get energy that lasts.

The Select Committee called particular attention to soft drinks: between 1960 and 1975 yearly soft drink consumption doubled from 109 12-ounce cans per capita to 221 cans.

Consequently, in reviewing the ways to cut the intake of refined sugar, the Dietary Goals suggest that "the most obvious item for general reduction is soft drinks. Total elimination of soft drinks from the diet, for many people, would bring at least half the recommended reduction in the consumption of such sugars."

At the beginning of this chapter, we pointed out that the average American eats two-thirds of a cup of sugar a day, much of it unwittingly. As you well know, you aren't sprinkling that much sugar on your food or even using it in cooking. In fact, we can neither see nor measure almost two-thirds of the sugar we eat — it is hidden away in the processed foods we bring home from the store. And with all the talk about the dangers of sugar, food manufacturers continue to load their products with sugar, "in large part to create unique products with a competitive edge. Just recently, for example, Nabisco introduced an Oreo cookie with double the amount of sugar filling," according to testimony before the Senate Select Committee.

Of course, you expect to find sugar in colas and cookies. You probably don't expect to find that 30 percent of a salad dressing is sugar. And even for the most conscientious label reader, there is virtually no way to tell just how much sugar a processed food contains. As of this writing, manufacturers are required only to list ingredients in order of predominance. If sugar is the first ingredient on the label, there is more sugar in that product than anything else — but you still don't know the quantity. Also, "sugar" may be only one of several forms of sugar in a particular food. Further down on the label, you may find corn syrup, honey, molasses, dextrose, maltose, fructose, lactose, glucose, or sucrose. The end product of all of these, in the digestive process, is exactly the same — glucose.

Nutrition and consumer groups have long been claiming that the only way for the purchaser to know how much sugar a product really has is for the label to list the percentage. Following a year of hearings around the country on food labeling, it looks as if this may be realized. Even so, you may have to add up all the different kinds of sugar to arrive at the true percentage, and even percentages can be misleading if liquid is added to the product in preparation. A cola drink, for example, has a lower *percentage* of sugar than does a bouillon cube, but it actually has much more sugar than the cup of bouillon you make by adding water to the cube.

In 1978, Consumers Union tested twenty-four common food products for their sugar content, measured in percentages. Here is what they found:

PRODUCT	PERCENT SUGAR
Cherry Jell-O	82.6
Coffee-Mate	65.4
Cremora	56.9
Hershey milk chocolate	51.4
Shake 'n Bake (Barbecue)	50.9
Sara Lee Chocolate Cake	35.9
Wishbone dressing (Russian)	30.2
Heinz ketchup	28.9
Quaker 100% Natural Cereal	23.9
Hamburger Helper	23.0
Wishbone dressing (French)	23.0
Sealtest chocolate ice cream	21.4
Cool Whip	21.0
Libby's peach halves	17.9
Shake 'n Bake (plain)	17.4
Wyler's beef-flavor bouillon cubes	14.8
Shake 'n Bake (Italian)	14.7
Dannon blueberry yogurt	13.7
Ritz crackers	11.8
Del Monte whole kernel corn	10.7
Skippy creamy peanut butter	9.2
Coca-Cola	8.8
Wishbone dressing (Italian)	7.3
Ragu spaghetti sauce	6.2

(In 1979, the Department of Agriculture tested the sugar content of sixty-two ready-to-eat cereals. See Chapter 13 for these ratings.)

To get away from white sugar and chemical additives,

more and more people are buying "natural" foods. This is fine so far as the additives go, but don't think that natural foods do not contain sugar. The Quaker 100% Natural Cereal in the preceding table is "naturally sweetened with brown sugar and honey" — to the tune of almost 24 percent. Are these natural sweeteners better for you than refined white sugar? The answer, unfortunately, is not really; all are converted identically in the body.

The brown sugar in that natural cereal (or in the box or plastic bag you buy in the store) is nothing but refined white sugar sprayed with molasses or caramelized white sugar. As for honey, as one nutritionist has said, the amount of nutrients contained in honey is enough to nourish a small bee. By all means eat honey if you like it, but remember that it counts as sugar.

Raw sugar is banned in this country because it contains bugs, dirt, mold, and bacteria. When it is refined enough to make it sanitary, but not pure, it is called turbinado sugar. As Consumer Reports states, the few additional nutrients in brown sugar or turbinado sugar "are so minuscule in quantity that for all practical purposes, they are worthless. The nutrients simply aren't there in the usable parts of the sugar cane and sugar beet plant to be refined out."

Alcohol

Chemically, alcohol is a substance very similar to sugar; nutritionally, in heavy drinkers, it presents problems above and beyond the other problems associated with alcoholism. Like sugar, alcohol is an empty-calorie food. It not only interferes with the absorption of several of the B vitamins in particular; alcohol further depresses the appetite for the foods that provide protein, minerals, and vitamins needed for its metabolism. Alcoholics are almost always seriously malnourished.

Some Ways to Reduce Sugar in the Diet

As in the case of all the Dietary Goals, the goal for sugar is based on a statistic — the amount of sugar consumed by the "average" American. Individuals are not average, and on the basis of your own diet, you may well find the statistic of an average consumption of one-third of a pound of sugar a day unbelievable. But consider this: for every person who eats less than that amount of sugar, there are others who eat more!

If you already consume very little sugar, these recommendations are already a part of your way of life. If you eat anywhere near the average, or more than the average, they should be taken very seriously.

1. Start young. Even though babies are apparently born with a sweet tooth, the way parents cater to it from infancy will affect not only their real teeth but their craving for sugar throughout life. Never buy a jar of baby food that has sugar on the label, don't sugar food to encourage a baby to eat it, and check the sugar content of cereals in Chapter 13.

2. Be *very* suspicious of food products heavily advertised on children's television shows. Don't fall for the television mother who sanctimoniously explains how careful she is about feeding her children snacks as she works up to handing them a Twinkie. Or that terrific mother who doses all the kids on the block with Kool-Aid.

3. Avoid all soft drinks. Substitute fruit juices, but look for the ones that are all juice, with no sugar added.

4. Read the labels on all packaged products. Where possible, select carefully among brands, but if all brands of a particular food product are high in sugar, ask yourself whether you really need that food at all. Nobody *needs* to help hamburgers along with a product that is one-quarter sugar or give the chicken a barbecue flavor with a coating that is more than half sugar.

5. Learn to satisfy your sweet tooth with a low-calorie, highly nutritious, naturally sweet food — fruit. Needless to say, don't add sugar to the fruit. If white grapefruit tastes too sour, try pink grapefruit instead. It is not only sweeter, it has more vitamin A.

6. Try to reduce overall your consumption of cookies and baked goods. When you make your own, don't follow the rec-

ipe for sugar — it's always too high — but see Chapter 23 for suggestions on how to cut down on the amount of sugar used in baking.

7. Remember that sugar is sugar, whether it's white, brown, or made by bees.

CHAPTER 7

Salt

TWENTY PERCENT of all Americans are susceptible to hypertension, the medical term for high blood pressure; among older people, the number at risk is 40 percent. Black people are twice as likely as whites to develop high blood pressure, usually earlier in life and in a more severe form.

The two dietary factors in hypertension are obesity — overweight people are much more likely to develop high blood pressure — and sodium, which we eat primarily in the form of sodium chloride, common table salt. There is also evidence that an imbalance between sodium and potassium (too much sodium, too little potassium) has an elevating effect on blood pressure.

Although some people apparently can eat virtually any amount of salt without ill effects, the evidence from both animal and epidemiological studies is that among those inherently susceptible, because of heredity, race, obesity, or other factors, salt intake is critically related to hypertension.

According to Dr. George Meneely and Dr. Harold Battarbee in *Present Knowledge in Nutrition*, "millions of children and youth are moving toward hypertension. Excess dietary sodium is clearly an adverse factor in some, if not most, people prone to hypertension. The evidence indicates that a systematic effort to reduce dietary sodium chloride intake and increase dietary potassium would . . . increase both duration and quality of life for millions of people."

How much salt do we eat? How much do we need? Some

simple mathematics clarifies the status of salt in our diet.

Sodium chloride, or salt, contains about 40 percent sodium, and it is the sodium that counts. Americans eat between 6000 and 18,000 milligrams of salt each day, although some researchers put the top number at 30,000 milligrams. Taking the more conservative figures and remembering that salt is 40 percent sodium, this means we consume between 2400 and 7200 milligrams of sodium daily.

The average human *need* for sodium is about 250 milligrams a day. In other words, we are eating somewhere between ten and twenty-nine times as much salt as our bodies require.

In the first edition of *Dietary Goals*, the Senate Select Committee on Nutrition recommended that we reduce salt intake to 3 grams. This was later revised upward to 5 grams — 5000 milligrams. This equals 2000 milligrams of sodium, or just what you get in one teaspoon of salt.

At first glance, this seems like a reasonable goal and one that should be easy to achieve. The hitch, however, is that a lot of the salt we consume comes from some place other than our own salt shakers, where we would be in a position to measure it. More than half the food we buy for home consumption is processed, and, according to Consumers Union, we eat about half our meals outside the home — which leaves much of our salt intake in the hands of food manufacturers and restaurants. A McDonald's cheeseburger with a side order of French fries and a chocolate milk shake add up to 1615 milligrams of sodium. If you put ketchup or mustard on the cheeseburger and salt on the potatoes, you will probably have exceeded the total Recommended Daily Allowance for 2000 milligrams of sodium.

Although sodium occurs naturally in most foods, the place it hits us hardest is in processed foods. There, if you read the labels, you will not only find salt but the word sodium as part of any one or more of a dozen different compounds, including sodium nitrate, sodium nitrite, and monosodium glutamate, three additives to avoid for other reasons. (See Chapter 10.)

Salt, according to *Dietary Goals*, "is added to processed

foods principally as a flavoring agent rather than a preservative. In some instances, it is the principal flavoring agent and may be used to mask other, less appealing, flavors."

Salt and sugar, the two principal additives to processed foods, are both used to enhance or alter taste. Unlike sugar, though, salt is a completely acquired taste. We aren't born with a liking for salt as we apparently are born with an innate predilection for sweet substances. For parents of infants and very young children, the easiest way to prevent hypertension through diet is to eliminate all salt from baby foods. If the word salt or sodium is on the label, don't buy the food; the salt was added to make it taste good to mother. For the same reason, you obviously should not add salt to the food you give a baby. How quickly we acquire our taste for salt can be seen in the typical habit of young children who put a little pile of salt on their plates and then dip their food into it. To most parents, this probably seems like a harmless way of getting a child to eat. It is anything but harmless.

As for those of us who, over many years, have become addicted to salt, how can we achieve our goal of one teaspoon a day? The Senate Select Committee suggests that we can do it by eliminating all salt from cooking, by not adding any at the table, and by avoiding foods with visible salt, such as potato chips and pretzels.

Unfortunately, this leaves all of our salt consumption to the discretion of the food manufacturers. Processed foods that are high in salt are probably low in potassium, the very substance needed to balance our sodium intake. These same foods are also likely to be rich in other additives, including sugar.

To see what happens to the balance between sodium and potassium in even lightly processed foods, compare these minerals in the following 100-gram portions of peas.

	SODIUM (MG)	POTASSIUM (MG)
Fresh peas	0.9	380
Frozen peas	100	160
Canned peas	230	180

As for the committee's injunction to avoid foods with visible salt, it's all right as far as it goes, which isn't far enough. A high salt content is not necessarily highly visible. It's probably no surprise to learn that an ounce of Mister Salty pretzel sticks contains about 892 milligrams of sodium, but would you expect one frozen meat loaf dinner to contain 2045? Even the McDonald's chocolate shake mentioned earlier had 329 milligrams of sodium — which is still less than half a cup of Jell-O instant chocolate pudding (486 milligrams). The salt you can't see can hurt you.

A better way to reduce salt intake to a safe level and eat palatable, healthier food is to reduce your sodium intake across the board — in cooking, at the table, and in processed foods. If the food you eat is tasty to begin with, there should be no need to add salt at the table. Still, since we are so in the habit of reaching for salt — sometimes even before tasting the food, a habit many cooks find downright insulting — you might try confining the salt shaker to the kitchen. It's a good way to keep children from developing the reflex salt habit. Instead, offer a little seasoning plate with lime or lemon wedges, a container of sesame seeds, some grated horseradish, and a pepper grinder.

In the beginning, if you are accustomed to liberal amounts of salt in and on your food, what you eat may, indeed, taste a little bland, but this will pass very soon, and you will discover that foods have flavors in and of themselves that are masked by added salt. In cooking, if you want added seasoning while learning to shake the salt habit, try sprinkling a little dill weed or celery seed (not celery salt) or garlic powder (again, not garlic salt) on vegetables or meat. Experiment with other herbs and spices, but remember that flavorings like soy sauce, especially, and ketchup or Worcestershire sauce are high in salt.

Since our sodium intake is increasingly determined by the food manufacturer, the habit of reading food labels can have a very significant effect on the amount of salt we consume in the course of a day. Unfortunately, the label won't tell you how many milligrams of salt are in the product, but it will give some clues as to the proportion in relation to other ingredients. Not all foods have to be labeled, and the whole procedure of food labeling has many problems (and is, as we write, under review); however, where food is labeled, the ingredients are listed in order of predominance. If you find salt in, say, third place, you can be sure that food is pretty salty. If you find a few other ingredients with the word sodium in them, it's even saltier. You may still want to buy the product, but at least you will do so with the knowledge that you had better cut down on your salt somewhere else. You may also discover that a similar food product with a lower amount of salt will serve your purpose just as well.

One word of caution: the individual who eats no processed foods at all should be sure to use some salt in cooking or at the table. *Some* sodium, the amount in about one-eighth of a teaspoon of salt, is necessary in the diet.

At the end of this chapter, we list the sodium content of a variety of natural and processed foods. While hardly a complete grocery list, it will give you an idea of the amount of sodium you can typically expect to find in different types of food products. As an enlightening experiment, you might want to look at some of the packages on your pantry shelf. One of us did just that and found a few surprises:

Kellogg's 40% Bran Flakes: Sugar was the second ingredient, salt the third.

MBT Instant Chicken Flavored Broth [*package*]: The first ingredient was salt, the third was monosodium glutamate, the fourth was sugar, and the fifth was dextrose (also sugar).

Campbell's Chicken Broth [*can*]: Here salt was the third ingredient, monosodium glutamate the fourth, and sugar the sixth.

The more "instant" the food, the more sugar, salt, and other additives it is likely to have. While even canned soups tend to be salty, they are a far better buy and more nutritional than "instant" products — and how many milliseconds do you really save for those extra milligrams of additives? Is heating up a can of liquid much harder than boiling water to add to a dry mix? Do you really expect the first

APPROXIMATE SODIUM CONTENT OF SOME
COMMON FOODS

FOOD	PORTION	SODIUM (MG)
Banana	1	1
Nabisco Shredded Wheat	1 ounce	1
Apple	1	2
Peanuts, unsalted	10	2
Orange juice	1 cup	2
Green beans*	1 cup	5
Kidney beans*	1 cup	6
Potato, baked	1	6
Del Monte canned peaches	1 cup	20
Birds Eye frozen broccoli	1 cup	30
Butter	1 tablespoon	46
Ice cream	1 cup	84
Whole milk	1 cup	122
Pillsbury chocolate chip cookies	3	130
Jif peanut butter	2 tablespoons	178
Heinz tomato ketchup	1 tablespoon	182
Pillsbury sugar cookies	3	210
Heinz mustard	1 tablespoon	213
Pepperidge Farm whole wheat bread	2 slices	214
Wonder potato chips	1 ounce	220
Hostess Twinkies	1	241
Oscar Mayer bacon	2 slices	285
Wonder white bread	2 slices	297
General Mills corn flakes	1 ounce	305
Del Monte tomato juice	4 ounces	320
Wishbone Italian salad dressing	1 tablespoon	362
Nabisco Wheat Thins	16 (1 ounce)	370
Kraft cheddar cheese, natural*	2 ounces	380
Oscar Mayer beef frankfurter	1	425
Del Monte tuna in oil	3 ounces	430
Oscar Mayer bologna	2 slices	450
Jell-O instant chocolate pudding	½ cup	486
Celeste frozen pizza	4 ounces	656

FOOD	PORTION	SODIUM (MG)
B & M baked red kidney beans *	1 cup	810
Kraft American cheese, processed *	2 ounces	890
Del Monte green beans, canned *	1 cup	925
Campbell's tomato soup	10 ounces	950
Hungry Jack pancakes, complete	3 four-inch	1150
Soy sauce	1 tablespoon	1320
Swanson frozen 3-course turkey dinner	1 (17 ounces)	1735
Dill pickle	1 large	1928

*Compare the sodium content of the natural versus the processed product.

three ingredients of onion soup to be sugar, salt, and monosodium glutamate (as in Croyden House Kosher Instant Onion Soup)?

One of the best ways to keep down the sodium in our diets is to eat natural foods. For the most part, these are the same foods that will help us meet all our Dietary Goals, not just the one for salt. Foods that are naturally low in sodium and generally high in potassium are fresh fruits and vegetables, dried beans, and whole grains.

If you are prone to indigestion and use over-the-counter remedies to relieve it, you may be adding to your salt load. As you can see, the amount of sodium varies widely among some of the more popular compounds.

DRUG	AVERAGE DOSE	SODIUM (MG)
Alka-Seltzer (blue)	2 tablets	1064
Bisodol powder	1 packet	1540
Bromo Seltzer	1.25 grams	717
Rolaids	2 tablets	100
Tums	2 tablets	40

CHAPTER 8

Vitamins and Minerals

FOODS ARE MADE UP of macronutrients (proteins, carbohydrates, and fats) and micronutrients (vitamins and minerals). Vitamins are organic substances that need the presence of inorganic minerals to be used effectively by the body. While specific vitamins and minerals do perform different functions, it is important not to ignore the interrelation of nutrients and their effects upon each other. For example:

• If you take large doses of one of the B vitamins when there is no indication that you have a deficiency in that vitamin, you could actually create a deficiency in the other B vitamins.
• A vitamin A supplement taken for a vitamin A deficiency will be useless if that deficiency — as can happen — was caused by a lack of vitamin E.
• Taking calcium pills to correct a calcium deficiency won't help if that deficiency is caused not by a lack of calcium but by a vitamin D deficiency — which is why milk is fortified with D.

Now that our love affair with vitamins has heated up into an affair with megavitamins — a space-age description of massive doses of vitamins taken not for therapeutic reasons but on the grounds that if a little is good, more is better — it is especially important to understand how complex and interrelated the functions of nutrients are. Even before Geritol hopped on the megavitamin bandwagon, it was advertising its iron supplement as containing "some very important vitamins, too." The implication, apparently, is that some vitamins aren't very important.

Actually, we don't know everything about all vitamins (some we may not know anything about), but that doesn't mean that they may not be important. Taking a vitamin pill "just to be sure" is good for the financial health of the manufacturer, but it is no guarantee that you'll get all the vitamins, known and unknown — to say nothing of other essential nutrients — that exist in a wide variety of natural foods. For, as deceptive as the implication that good nutritional health can be achieved through vitamin pills is the even more insidious idea that you can get all your daily food needs in such things as a nutrition bar, a synthetic combination of sugar, chemical additives, and "100 percent" of the daily requirement for fourteen vitamins. *Far* better to eat a real candy bar and know you have to fill your nutritional needs with other food than to fool yourself into thinking that a piece of "nutrition" chocolate or "total" cereal is doing the job. It isn't.

Perhaps the most important thing to remember when you take vitamin pills is the word *supplement*. Vitamin pills, correctly used, are not a replacement for food but a supplement to a diet that is low in one or more essential nutrients. Similarly, when you eat food "fortified" with vitamins and minerals, the bottom line is whether the food is good to begin with. Adding vitamin D to milk makes it possible for the body to utilize the calcium in the milk, but adding vitamins to sugar doesn't turn sugar into a health food.

Although serious vitamin and mineral deficiencies are not a problem for the average American, the increased consumption of processed vegetables and fruits and refined grain products has had an effect on the amount of certain vitamins and minerals we get from our food. As recently as 1959, most of the fruits and vegetables we ate were in the form of fresh produce. By 1971, a mere twelve years later, the proportion had shifted, and more than half of these foods were being consumed as processed produce. Since the proportion of processed foods has continued to rise, these percentages would be considerably higher today. A Department of Agriculture report published in 1972 found that nutrient "availability" from vegetables had declined both as a result of the switch toward processed foods and the shift away from potatoes, dark green and yellow vegetables, dry beans and peas, and grain products.

In *Dietary Goals*, the Select Committee on Nutrition urges that we shift the balance back to more fresh fruits and vegetables. While we know a lot about the nutritional impact of freezing, canning, and other processing, "this knowledge is not held for all nutrients, all foods, or all processes. Furthermore, it is important to understand what constitutes food value. Out of 50 known nutrients, Recommended Dietary Allowances* have been set for only 17. In addition, there is no definitive evidence that food composition described solely in terms of all known nutrients would be an accurate measure of total food value."

While it is possible to restore certain nutrients through fortification, it is doubtful, the report states, that the numbers and balance in the fresh form can ever be duplicated. What is true for processed fruits and vegetables is also true for grain products. "In bread, as with other foods undergoing processing, there is danger that as the degree of

---

* RDA versus U.S. RDA. To the consumer, this is a distinction without a difference. The RDAs (Recommended *Dietary* Allowances) are established by the Food and Nutrition Board of the National Academy of Sciences. Based on available scientific knowledge, the board considers these to be the levels of intake of essential nutrients that will meet the known nutritional needs of practically all healthy people. The U.S. RDAs (Recommended *Daily* Allowances) are figures derived from the RDAs by the Food and Drug Administration (FDA) as standards for nutritional labeling.

For the most part the figures are the same. A notable exception is protein, where the FDA takes into consideration the quality of the protein in the product and whether it is a complete protein, as in meat and dairy foods, or an incomplete protein, as in most plant foods. For example, a can of beef stew and a can of kidney beans may contain the same amount of protein. This total amount is listed in the left-hand column on the label. However, since the meat protein is of higher quality than the bean protein, this difference is accounted for in the right-hand column of the label, which tells what *percentage* of the U.S. RDA for protein the product contains. When you read labels, concentrate on the right-hand column.

processing increases, nutrients, known and unknown, are removed or altered in ways not currently understood."

With some exceptions, which are noted in this chapter, a diet based on the Dietary Goals will provide an adequate amount of all the vitamins and minerals the body needs. Whether you take vitamin or mineral supplements is, of course, up to you, but if you keep them in the house, keep them away from children. Of the 4000 cases of vitamin poisoning reported each year to the National Clearinghouse for Poison Control Centers, 3200 involve children. Bottles of children's vitamins should be kept away from children too. A four-year-old Kansas boy who swallowed forty tablets of his own pills spent two days in intensive care suffering from vitamin A and iron poisoning.

Vitamins

Under certain circumstances and at certain times of life, deficiencies in specific vitamins can be quite common. These are discussed under the vitamins in question, but in general, people who fall into any of the following categories should be aware of the possibility of a general or specific vitamin deficiency:

• Anyone who is on a diet.
• Pregnant women and nursing mothers.
• Heavy smokers, who require additional vitamin C.
• Heavy drinkers, who are generally deficient in the B vitamins.
• Elderly people, who are likely to be deficient in both vitamin C and the B vitamins.
• People taking oral contraceptives or cortisone drugs, both of which create a vitamin B_6 deficiency.

Vitamin A (Carotene)

Vitamin A occurs only in animal foods. However, the body transforms carotene, which occurs in vegetables, into vitamin A.

Vitamin A is essential for the proper development of skin and mucous membranes and the growth of bones and tooth enamel in children. The first sign of a deficiency is night blindness. Other indications of deficiency are rough dry skin, nails, and hair. Although carrots probably won't give you curly hair, as our mothers promised us, they can make it nice and shiny.

Vitamin A is easy to come by in the food supply, and it is unlikely that anyone who eats reasonably well will have a deficiency, especially since it is soluble in fats and can be stored in the body for several months. However, vitamin A is destroyed if there is a vitamin E deficiency, and it also needs vitamin D to be properly absorbed. Milk should be fortified with both vitamin A and D.

In excess doses vitamin A is toxic, and no vitamin capsule may contain more than 10,000 International Units (IU) except by prescription. Unfortunately, there is nothing to stop a vitamin-happy consumer from taking more than one tablet a day.

On the other hand, as long as you can control your craving for polar bear liver, there is virtually no way to overdose on vitamin A in foods, since much of that vitamin is ingested in the form of carotene, and carotene is not toxic in any quantity. The worst that could happen is that your hands might turn temporarily yellow, proof that the body is not converting the overload to vitamin A.

The best sources of vitamin A are liver and fish liver oils. Good sources are butter, cheese, eggs, and milk. Carotene is plentiful since it occurs in all the yellow and orange vegetables and in leafy greens. The darker the orange or green color, the more carotene the vegetable contains. Carotene is also used as a food coloring — a perfectly safe one, naturally.

U.S. RDA FOR VITAMIN A

Infants	1500 IU
Children under 4	2500
Adults and children over 4	5000
Pregnant or lactating women	8000

The RDAs for vitamin A are based on weight and computed on the assumption that people will get half their requirements from vitamin A itself and half from carotene. Vegetarians who don't eat any dairy products get only carotene and should eat more than the recommended amount.

Since some vitamin A is destroyed in cooking, cook foods briefly in a minimum amount of water, and save the water. This vitamin is also destroyed by light.

The amount of vitamin A or carotene in foods is quite variable, depending on the season, the soil, the maturity of the plant, and other factors including storage and preparation. The high vitamin A content in the following foods are approximate.

Calf liver, 2 ounces	30,280 IU
Dandelion greens, 1 cup cooked	21,060
Sweet potato, canned, 1 cup	17,000
Carrots, 1 cup cooked	15,220
Pumpkin, canned, 1 cup	14,590
Spinach, 1 cup cooked	14,580
Collard greens, 1 cup cooked	10,260
Sweet potato, 1 baked	8,910
Winter squash, 1 cup baked	8,610
Turnip greens, 1 cup cooked	8,270
Kale, 1 cup cooked	8,140
Beet greens, 1 cup cooked	7,400
Cantaloupe, ½ medium	6,540
Broccoli, 1 stalk cooked	4,500

Many other fruits and vegetables are good sources of vitamin A, including red peppers, asparagus, tomatoes, nectarines, apricots, pink grapefruit, and romaine lettuce. Dairy sources include eggs, butter or margarine, cheddar cheese, and whole milk.

B Vitamins

These are a group of water soluble vitamins that cannot be stored in the body and must be replenished regularly. Although Americans are highly unlikely to incur the serious

forms of vitamin B deficiency — pellagra, beriberi, or pernicious anemia — mild deficiencies can be quite common in
a diet that is high in refined flours and sugar. While enrichment replaces some of the B vitamins lost in milling, it
doesn't replace them all. Sugar is the villain on a number of
counts. The need for certain of the B vitamins increases with
the amount of carbohydrates you eat, but whereas other carbohydrates contribute B vitamins, sugar only increases the
need for them without adding any to the pool. Sugar also
reduces the desire for foods that have B vitamins. Certain
medications also increase the need for specific B vitamins.

Except for B_{12}, which is found only in animal foods, the
other B vitamins occur in the same foods in varying
amounts. Foods that offer plenty of B_1 and B_2 are likely to be
the ones that have all the B vitamins (except for B_6 and B_{12})
you need. Although each of the B vitamins has a separate
function, they are interdependent, and a deficiency in one
probably means a deficiency in the others. Conversely, an
excess in one will increase the need for the others and cause
a deficiency if that need is not met. That's why people who
take supplementary doses of a single B vitamin could actually be inviting a vitamin B deficiency.

Because B_{12} occurs only in animal foods, vegetarians who
do not eat dairy products require a vitamin B_{12} supplement.

VITAMIN B_1 (THIAMIN)

Thiamin acts to convert protein and carbohydrates into
energy, and the need for this vitamin increases with the total
amount of calories you eat, particularly calories from carbohydrates. The brain and the central nervous system are
particularly susceptible to thiamin deficiency, which first
shows up as loss of stamina, depression, irritability, and lack
of concentration.

In the Orient, where rice is a staple of the diet, beriberi be-
came endemic when polished white rice, imported by west-
erners, replaced whole grain rice in the diet. In the United
States, the possibility of this kind of deficiency has been

reduced by enrichment of refined flours. However, as noted earlier, sugar, which contains no vitamins but creates an increased need for thiamin and certain other B vitamins, is a major cause of mild thiamin deficiency in this country. Also, although whole grain and enriched breads contain thiamin, toasting partially destroys this vitamin.

The adult U.S. RDA for thiamin is 1.5 mg.

Thiamin is found in many foods. Some of the best sources are the following:

Brewer's yeast, 1 tablespoon	1.2 mg
Pork, 2 ounces	.63
Pinto beans, 1 cup cooked	.51
Peas, 1 cup cooked	.45
Wheat germ, ¼ cup toasted	.44
Sunflower seeds, 2 tablespoons hulled	.36
Black beans, 1 cup cooked	.35
Lima beans, 1 cup cooked	.31
Split peas, 1 cup cooked	.30
Spinach, 1 cup cooked	.25
Orange, 1 large	.24
Asparagus, 1 cup cooked	.23
Calf liver, 3 ounces cooked	.22

Other sources are oatmeal, brown rice, whole wheat bread, sesame seeds, nuts, meats, yams, broccoli, and other vegetables.

VITAMIN B_2 (RIBOFLAVIN)

Milk and milk products are the best sources in our diets of riboflavin, whose primary function is the metabolism of protein. The best single source is liver — two ounces of beef liver provide a full day's requirement. Other good B_2 foods are meat, whole grains, and enriched breads and cereals.

Since riboflavin is easily destroyed by light, the milk we buy today in cartons or plastic bottles is considerably richer in this vitamin than it was in the good old days when the milkman left it on the back porch. Naturally, you will store milk and meat products in the refrigerator, but remember to keep bread and grains in light-proof containers too.

The adult U.S. RDA for riboflavin is 1.7 mg.

The best dairy sources are cottage cheese, low-fat milk, yogurt, and whole milk. The best vegetables are collard greens, broccoli, mushrooms, winter squash, asparagus, and spinach. Remember, ripe vegetables should be stored in the refrigerator.

NIACIN

For reasons too complicated to attempt to explain here, even the Food and Nutrition Board which sets the RDAs admits that estimating the actual niacin requirements is difficult. To allow for a lot of variables, the Recommended Dietary Allowance is probably much higher than is actually necessary. The U.S. RDA for adults is 20 mg.

The best sources of niacin are lean meats, fish, and poultry (white meat of chicken has twice as much as the dark meat); cottage cheese, whole grains and enriched cereals and breads; all kinds of peas and beans, peanuts, and leafy green vegetables.

FOLIC ACID (FOLACIN)

This B vitamin is widespread in foods, especially liver, leafy vegetables, yeast, and some fruits. However, it is not clearly known to what extent the vitamin is absorbed from food.

Folacin is of primary importance to pregnant women, since the need for this vitamin increases markedly in pregnancy and fetal damage has been linked to a deficiency. The U.S. RDA for pregnant and lactating women is 0.8 mg, twice the 0.4 mg for adults.

A vitamin supplement will correct this deficiency. The amount of folacin that may be added to any vitamin pill is 0.1 mg. Since the synthetic vitamin is four times as strong as the folacin in food, this is equal to the *extra* amount required for pregnancy. The reason for placing a legal limit on this vitamin supplement is that it can hide the symptoms of a vitamin B_{12} deficiency.

VITAMIN B_6 (PYRIDOXINE, PYRIDOXAL, PYRIDOXAMINE)

The problems of determining RDAs for B_6 are, according to the Food and Nutrition Board, "considerably different from those for most of the other vitamins for which allowances have been established, because there is no area in the world where a deficiency has been clearly related to poor nutrition. However, a B_6 deficiency has been implicated in an extraordinary number of seemingly unrelated conditions, but involving large numbers of individuals, and so in spite of lack of information on the exact need for this vitamin or even its availability in food, RDAs have been established for B_6."

Several groups of people — pregnant women, women taking oral contraceptives, and people taking cortisone — should be particularly careful to ensure that they are getting enough B_6. The requirement for this vitamin is also related to the amount of protein in the diet — the more protein you eat, the more pyridoxine you need. (See Chapter 4.)

The U.S. RDA for B_6 for adults is 2 mg; for pregnant and lactating women it is 2.5 mg. According to the Food and Nutrition Board, however, the amount of B_6 needed by women taking oral steroid contraceptives appears to be far greater than can be supplied in a normal diet. So if you are on the Pill, take a vitamin pill.

The best sources of B_6 are wheat germ, meat, liver, whole grain cereals, soybeans, peanuts, and corn. This is one of the vitamins removed in milling that is *not* replaced in enriched bread. Vitamin B_6 is destroyed by heat; meat that is cooked for a long time or under high heat may lose up to 50 percent of the vitamin. So do canned foods.

B $_{12}$ (COBALAMIN)

The extreme form of vitamin B$_{12}$ deficiency is pernicious anemia, which is caused by an inability to absorb B$_{12}$. For normal individuals even mild deficiencies are highly unlikely except for vegetarians who eat no animal products at all. Since B$_{12}$ does not occur in plant foods, vegan vegetarians require a supplement.

In large amounts, B$_{12}$ is found in organ meats such as liver and in shellfish such as clams and oysters — all high-cholesterol foods. It occurs in smaller amounts in meat, fish, poultry, eggs, and dairy products.

There is a considerable difference of opinion as to the amount of B$_{12}$ necessary to the body. Dr. Victor Herbert, professor of pathology and professor of medicine at Columbia University College of Physicians and Surgeons, writes in *Present Knowledge in Nutrition* that "the Food and Agriculture Organization/World Health Organization recommends a daily intake of 2 μg [micrograms] of vitamin B$_{12}$ for the normal adult, allowing a substantial margin above normal physiological requirements."

The Food and Nutrition Board of the National Academy of Sciences recommends a slightly higher intake — 3 micrograms for adults and 4 for pregnant and lactating women. But the Food and Drug Administration recommends a much higher allowance — 6 micrograms for adults and 8 for pregnant and lactating women.

As discussed earlier, large amounts of a folic acid supplement may mask a vitamin B$_{12}$ deficiency. And large doses of vitamin C increase the need for vitamin B$_{12}$. According to Dr. Herbert, these large doses of vitamin C can destroy between 50 and 95 percent of the B$_{12}$ in a meal.

BIOTIN

Not very much is known about this B vitamin except that apparently the only way you can cause a biotin deficiency is by eating eight or more raw egg whites every day. Not likely. Since biotin is manufactured by the body as well as ingested in food, the human daily requirement for the vitamin is not known.

PANTOTHENIC ACID

Panto means everywhere, and this B vitamin is almost universally present in plant as well as animal tissues and is also manufactured by the body. Marginal deficiencies, where they are present, are usually found in connection with other vitamin B deficiencies.

The U.S. RDA for pantothenic acid is 10 mg.

Vitamin C (Ascorbic Acid)

As far back as 1747, a surgeon's mate on an English ship conducted an experiment in which he proved that citrus fruits could prevent and cure scurvy. A half century later, the Royal Navy ordered that every man on its ships be administered an ounce of lime juice every day. So successful was vitamin C in wiping out scurvy that it is often credited with having done as much as Lord Nelson in breaking the power of Napoleon. Vitamin C was isolated and named in 1933.

Uncontroversially, vitamin C is known to help hold body cells together, strengthen blood vessels, help heal wounds, help in tooth and bone formation, and help in resistance to infection. Controversially, it either does or does not help prevent or cure the common cold.

While we do not intend here to line up with or against Linus Pauling, the foremost advocate of vitamin C megadoses, some caution is advisable. Side effects have been noted with doses of several grams daily, including severe diarrhea, kidney stones, and the inability to test accurately for diabetes. Research has also shown that large doses of vitamin C can destroy between 50 and 95 percent of the vitamin B_{12} in a meal. In general, there is evidence that vitamin C has some effect on colds, but there are still questions about the safety of massive doses. Although they may be safe for some people, are they safe for everyone?

Outside of the therapeutic level, vitamin C is, of course, essential in the diet. Since it is water-soluble and not stored in the body, it needs to be replenished daily. Vitamin C is extremely easy to come by in the food supply. Because it is best preserved in an acid environment, citrus fruits, even canned ones, are excellent sources. In smaller but significant amounts, C is found in other fruits, tomatoes, potatoes, and leafy green vegetables. It is an unstable vitamin, though, and easily destroyed by oxidation. (See Chapter 11 on ways to preserve vitamin C in foods.)

The vitamin C content of fruits and vegetables is variable, depending in part on climate, season, the amount of sun they get, and other factors including preparation.

The U.S. RDA for adults is 60 mg. Although the following amounts are approximate, all of these foods are excellent sources of this vitamin.

Broccoli, 1 stalk cooked	160 mg
Sweet red pepper, 1 raw	150
Brussels sprouts, 8 cooked	140
Orange juice, 1 cup	120
Kale, 1 cup cooked	100
Green pepper, 1 raw	94
Cantaloupe, ½ medium	90
Strawberries, 1 cup	88
Cauliflower, 1 cup cooked	69
Orange, 1 medium	66
Grapefruit, ½ medium	54
Spinach, 1 cup cooked	50
Cabbage, 1 cup cooked	48

Other fruits, berries, and vegetables, both cooked and uncooked, are very good sources of vitamin C.

Vitamin D

Vitamin D is essential to the proper absorption of calcium; in its absence children get rickets and adults osteomalacia. Although it is sometimes called the sunshine vitamin because the body can manufacture vitamin D in the presence of sunlight, this source is not really reliable, since there are too many variables, including weather and skin pigmentation. In dark-skinned people, as much as 95 percent of the sun's rays may be screened out.

Like vitamin A, the other major fat-soluble vitamin, D is stored in the body and does not have to be replenished daily. Taken in excess quantities in synthetic form, it can become toxic; the limit allowed in any one vitamin pill is 400 IU, which is the U.S. RDA for all people. Fish liver oils and fortified milk are the only major food sources of D.

Vitamin E

Vitamin E is another fat-soluble vitamin that is stored in the body and does not have to be replaced every day. Its chief function is as an antioxidant; it inhibits other substances from combining with oxygen and thus acts as a preservative.

The need for E increases with an increased consumption of polyunsaturated fats. However, most polyunsaturated fats have adequate amounts of this vitamin, so the increased need is automatically fulfilled. (Some vegetable-oil margarines contain thirteen times as much vitamin E as butter.)

Will vitamin E make hair grow? cure your skin problems? ease arthritis pain? prevent aging? make you sexually young? prevent ulcers? These are just a few of the miracle claims for megadoses of this vitamin — none of which, according to the FDA, has ever been proved in scientific studies in humans. On the other hand, although E is fat-soluble, the FDA has not found that large doses are toxic. Nevertheless, among individuals, megadoses have led to headaches, fatigue, nausea, and weakness.

The U.S. RDA for infants is 5 IU; for adult women, 2–25 IU; for men and pregnant and nursing mothers, 30 IU.

The best sources of vitamin E are vegetable oils, margarine, wheat germ, whole grains, liver, dried beans, and leafy green vegetables.

Vitamin K

There is no RDA for vitamin K, the antihemorrhagic agent, since deficiencies do not exist except in rare instances, in which case it is prescribed therapeutically. Excessive use of vitamin K supplements can be toxic.

The best sources of this vitamin are spinach, cabbage, cauliflower, and liver. The vitamin is also manufactured in the body.

Minerals

Minerals have two general functions in the body: building and regulating. The building function affects the skeleton and all soft tissues. The regulating functions affect a variety of systems including the heartbeat, blood clotting, and the transport of oxygen from the lungs to the tissues.

Some minerals are needed in relatively large amounts, notably calcium and phosphorus, the primary materials of bones and teeth, but also sodium, potassium, chlorine, magnesium, and sulfur. In tiny quantities, the important trace minerals are iron, manganese, copper, iodine, zinc, cobalt, fluorine, selenium, and possibly others.

A few minerals — lead, mercury, and cadmium — are dangerous. But even "good" minerals can be dangerous in larger than normal amounts. The excessive amount of sodium that we eat in salt (sodium chloride) is implicated in high blood pressure. Some scientists believe that the problem is not just too much sodium but too little potassium in relation to the sodium. However, if you were to try to correct this imbalance by eating your entire daily requirement of potassium in one concentrated dose, you could become seriously ill. Each year, many children are hospitalized, and some die, as the result of swallowing a quantity of iron supplement pills. These accidental poisonings can be prevented by keeping all pills away from children. There is a hazard for adults too. Some minerals can cause adverse health effects if pills containing as little as twice the normal dose are taken.

Taking too much of one mineral may upset the balance and function of other minerals in the body. According to the FDA, excess mineral intake can contribute to such health problems as anemia, bone demineralization, neurological disease, and fetal abnormalities. The risks are greatest for young children, pregnant women, nursing mothers, the elderly, and people with inadequate diets or a chronic disease.

Because there are things we do not know about the function of minerals in the body, particularly the trace minerals, the FDA recommends that people who take mineral supplements should not use them in amounts greatly in excess of the known requirements. In other words, no megadoses.

U.S. RDAs have been set for only seven minerals. This doesn't mean that the other minerals are not important, but only that there is not adequate information on which to set an allowance.

Macrominerals

CALCIUM

Almost all of the two or three pounds of calcium we carry around is in our bones and teeth. Although growing children and pregnant and lactating women have the greatest need for calcium, all people, including the elderly, need calcium in their diets throughout their lives.

Calcium deficiencies can be caused by other things than a lack of calcium in the diet. Any one of the following three factors can have a detrimental effect on the way calcium is used.

1. A vitamin D deficiency.
2. An imbalance between calcium and phosphorus. Too little or too much phosphorus — the latter is more likely — will inhibit the body's utilization of calcium.
3. Excessive protein intake, which also lowers the amount of calcium the body can absorb. People who eat a lot of meat (which is not only rich in protein but also in phosphorus and contains no calcium) should balance their diets with calcium-rich foods.

The U.S. RDA for calcium is 0.8 of a gram (800 mg) for children under 4; 1 gram for older children and adults, and 1.3 grams for pregnant and lactating women.

Milk, yogurt, and cheese are excellent sources of calcium. So are sardines, leafy green vegetables (with the exception of spinach, chard, sorrel, and parsley), and dried peas and beans. Meat, grains, and nuts do not provide significant amounts of calcium.

PHOSPHORUS

Phosphorus is present in bones and teeth in nearly the same amount as calcium and is also an important part of all tissues in the body. It is so widely available in foods, including meat, poultry, fish, eggs, and whole grains, that no one will have trouble obtaining a sufficient amount in the diet.

The problem, as mentioned earlier, is much more likely to be that of too much phosphorus, particularly in a meat-based diet. In addition to the natural phosphorus in foods, phosphates are used as preservatives in many processed foods.

SODIUM AND CHLORIDE

Although these two minerals are eaten in the form of sodium chloride (table salt), they have separate functions. The amount of chloride in our diets follows the amount of sodium, which is generally too high. Nevertheless, too much chloride doesn't seem to be a problem, as too much sodium definitely is. Please read about sodium in Chapter 7.

POTASSIUM

With sodium, potassium helps to regulate the balance and volume of body fluids. Since potassium is abundant in almost all plant and animal foods, a deficiency is very uncommon if at least some fresh food is eaten. One can result from prolonged diarrhea or from the use of diuretic drugs. Deficiencies have also been found in children on extremely inadequate protein diets.

MAGNESIUM

Magnesium is found in all body tissues, but principally in the bones. It is an essential part of many enzyme systems that are important in maintaining electrical potential in nerves and muscle membranes.

Although observable magnesium deficiency does not occur except in connection with other serious diseases involving total malnutrition (such as chronic alcoholism and childhood malnutrition), this is not to say that our dietary magnesium can be taken for granted.

In the past fifty years or so, the amount of magnesium in the average diet has dropped by one-fifth. The reasons for this quite drastic decline become apparent when you realize that the richest dietary sources of magnesium are whole grains, fresh leafy vegetables, and dried beans — especially the last. Magnesium is lost when flour is refined and is not replaced in the so-called enrichment process. Since it is soluble in water, canned or cooked vegetables have lower amounts of magnesium than raw unless the water is used. And, of course, dried beans are not a staple of the average diet. There is also some evidence that food grown in chemically fertilized soil has reduced magnesium content.

The Food and Nutrition Board of the National Academy of Sciences reports that estimates of the amount of magnesium required by adult men range from a low of 200 mg a day to a high of 700 mg. It is interesting to note that one of the authorities quoted raised his own estimate of 300 mg (in 1964) to 700 mg (in 1971). In 1980 the Food and Nutritional Board set an RDA of 300 mg for women and 350 mg for men (400 mg for 15 to 18 year olds), and 450 mg for pregnant and lactating women. It says that "the requirements . . . during pregnancy and lactation have received little attention recently."

The FDA, however, is more cautious — or more concerned. This is one of the rare instances where the U.S. RDA differs from the standards set by the Food and Nutrition Board. The

U.S. RDA for magnesium is 200 mg for children under 4, 400 mg for older children and adults, and 450 mg for pregnant or lactating women.

Mild magnesium deficiencies show up as muscle weakness and nervous irritability. Prolonged deficiency can produce irregular heartbeats, tremors, leg cramps, and muscle twitching. Alcoholics and patients on diuretics for a long time are prone to magnesium deficiency. People whose diets are restricted in variety and based on refined and processed foods may well have marginal deficiencies.

The best sources of magnesium are wheat germ, whole wheat flour, and dried beans, especially soybeans. Other very good sources are leafy greens — beet greens, spinach, Swiss chard, turnip greens, and collards. Potatoes and peas and most other vegetables have magnesium in rather smaller amounts.

Trace Minerals

Trace minerals are those needed by the body in tiny amounts. Of the seventeen known to have some biological function in humans, only a few are understood well enough to be evaluated for human nutrition. These are fluorine, chromium, manganese, iron, cobalt, copper, zinc, selenium, molybdenum, and iodine. Of these, U.S. RDAs have been set for only four — iron, iodine, zinc, and copper.

"Nutritional problems associated with deficient intake of iron, fluorine, and iodine are known to exist within the United States," according to the Food and Nutrition Board, which adds that "recent evidence suggests that intakes of zinc and chromium may be marginal in some segments of the population."

And studies by a Department of Agriculture scientist suggest that diets low in copper may raise the level of plasma cholesterol even where dietary cholesterol is reduced. Experimental rats fed a low-copper diet for six months had cholesterol concentrations in their blood that were 130 percent greater than the concentration in control rats. Dr. Leslie M. Klevay also reported that a study of twenty diets prepared from ordinary foods by professional nutritionists in hospitals and educational institutions (and "presumed to give good nourishment") showed that only two of the twenty contained the U.S. RDA of 2 mg of copper a day.

It is, of course, debatable whether institutional diets can be said to give good nutrition. However, the average individual diet is frequently no better, unfortunately.

IRON

Iron deficiencies are common among certain groups of people, and not many foods contain iron in usable amounts. However, merely because you do not meet your RDA for iron is not proof that you need an iron supplement. The U.S. RDA is set very high to protect individuals who need a lot of iron, and many people can get by with less.

In the normal individual, iron absorption is modified according to need, but some people do require supplementary iron. Self-diagnosis, in response to advertising that promotes iron supplements as a cure for listlessness or tiredness, is foolhardy and can be useless, even dangerous. Those symptoms can signal any one of a number of conditions other than iron anemia. In fact, people with mild anemia rarely know they have it until it is discovered in a blood test. Besides, not all anemia is *iron* anemia. For adult men and postmenopausal women, iron supplements are almost always unnecessary — since the average diet does contain enough iron in their cases — and potentially harmful because they could cover up and delay the diagnosis of gastrointestinal cancer, which sometimes first shows up as an iron-deficiency anemia.

Pregnant women, more likely than not, need more iron than they can get in food or that they have stored up. A doctor should prescribe the amount of supplementation needed.

Young children, from six months to five years, are quite likely to have an iron-deficiency anemia because of their rapid growth. Though some cereals and other foods are now enriched with iron, your pediatrician may recommend an iron supplement.

Nonpregnant women of childbearing age are the primary target for iron-supplement advertising because the fact is that 95 percent of them don't get anywhere near their recommended amount of 18 mg in their food. But this is the case where those RDAs are set abnormally high for most people in order to protect the ones who need it. Only about one in ten women in this group actually do have an iron deficiency. They are likely to be women who menstruate heavily or have diets low in iron.

Adolescent girls who are menstruating and also growing quickly and may, in addition, subsist on a junk-food diet are high risks for iron-deficiency anemia.

In all of these cases, the only way to tell whether you are anemic is to have a blood test.

Good sources of iron in the food supply are not plentiful. The most usable iron comes from meat, particularly liver. Meat not only supplies the "best" iron; it enables the body to absorb the iron in other kinds of foods. Citrus fruits also help in absorption. Iron is also present in shellfish, beans, peas, spinach, dried fruits, eggs, whole grain cereals, and enriched bread, but it is not in a chemical form that is particularly available to the body as is the iron in meat. Milk is a poor source of iron.

To compound the difficulty of assessing the body's needs, we absorb iron at very uneven and at times inefficient rates. Normal, healthy people may absorb only 5 percent of the iron in their diets; yet if there is a state of depletion in the body, the rate can rise to 30 percent. Once absorbed, it is stored in the body to be used over and over again for some time. The only way that iron can be lost in large amounts is through bleeding, as in menstruation and hemorrhaging, and in pregnant women who transfer large amounts of iron to the fetus and the placenta.

On the face of it, a vegetarian would seem to be a candidate for iron-deficiency anemia and so would the person who follows the Dietary Goals by cutting down on such high-cholesterol foods as liver and shellfish and meat.

For most people, good eating habits and a wide selection of unprocessed foods throughout life will go a long way to ensure an adequate amount of iron, except under abnormal circumstances. The prevalence of iron-deficiency anemia is testimony to the fact that most of us do not eat very well.

The U.S. RDA for iron is 10 mg for children under 4 and 18 mg for everyone else. For male adults and postmenopausal females, 18 mg is considerably higher than the recommendation of the Food and Nutrition Board, which holds that 10 mg a day is plenty.

The board also points out that the adult woman on a balanced diet will consume about 9–12 mg of iron from the food supply, and that a supplement will be needed to reach the 18 mg requirement. It admittedly has set the allowance very high to cover individuals who need it. Once again, the only way to tell whether you are one of those individuals is to have a blood test.

Note: One way to increase the amount of iron you eat is to use iron pots for cooking, especially for cooking stews and other foods that require a long cooking time. You will lose vitamin C by cooking in an iron pot, but long cooking isn't good for vitamin C anyway, and this vitamin is also much easier to find in food than iron.

ZINC

The discovery in recent years of the human need for zinc serves as an exemplar of the importance of ongoing identification of nutrients and the consequent need for eating a wide range of natural foods.

Zinc deficiency symptoms were identified only in 1963, when it was established that zinc was indeed a dietary essential for man. Though its exact role in vital bodily functions is still being studied, zinc is known to be a necessary component in DNA, RNA, and protein metabolism. The reproductive system particularly can be profoundly affected by zinc deficiency; in the Middle and Near East it has resulted in stunted growth and delayed sexual maturation, according to studies of groups of boys and girls. There the primary cause appeared to be a diet high in cereals, to the exclusion of other foods. Marginal zinc deficiency has appeared in the United States, where it was identified in children in Colorado.

With adults, it is often seen in connection with patients already suffering from alcoholism and/or cirrhosis of the liver and with illnesses as varied as sickle cell anemia, chronic kidney disease, or severe trauma. Like other mineral elements, a deficiency can occur in hospitalized patients, particularly those receiving intravenous feeding.

The U.S. RDA has recently been set at 15 mg for adults. The best sources are in meat, liver, shellfish (particularly oysters), and eggs, all foods that are also high in cholesterol. While whole grains and other plant foods, including beans and spinach, also contain zinc, the amount will be reduced if the plants are grown in zinc-poor soil.

Scientists know that for rats zinc, like iron, is more available from animal products, and the assumption is that it may be true for humans as well. However, there is no reason to believe that a widely based diet, such as the Dietary Goals recommend, could not adequately supply the small amount of zinc needed by normal individuals.

IODINE

Iodine is required in extremely small amounts, but the normal function of the thyroid gland depends on an adequate supply. Deficiencies, in the form of goiters, were common in certain inland areas of the United States, where the soil contains little iodine, until 1924, when iodized salt was introduced. Although iodization of salt is not mandatory, under an FDA regulation salt that is *not* iodized must be so labeled. For safety, especially if you live inland, be sure to buy iodized salt.

If anything, with the amount of salt we eat and the amount of iodine in other forms used in dough conditioners, antiseptics in dairy products, and other iodine additives, we may be eating an excessive amount. Although it doesn't appear to be a problem, too much iodine in the body could affect the thyroid in the same way as too little. There's no reason to try to increase the amount of iodine in your diet by eating dried seaweed or taking iodine tablets, and it might be dangerous.

In addition to iodized salt, iodine is found in all food from the sea. The U.S. RDA for iodine is an easily secured 150 *micro*grams.

FLUORINE

Fluorine is found in small and varying amounts in soil, plants, animals, and water. It is primarily available (or not available) in the water supply. In all communities where the water supply has been fluoridated, cavities in children have been reduced by more than 50 percent. In addition, there is now evidence that fluorine helps retain the calcium in the bones of old people; far fewer cases of osteoporosis are found in old people living in areas where fluorine has been added to the water. Research with animals has shown fluorine effective in accelerating wound healing as well as assisting in the body's iron absorption.

Because there is so little reliable fluorine in food — tea is a fair source and so are small fish eaten with their bones — the Food and Nutrition Board recommends fluoridation of the water supply, where the water is lacking in fluorine, as the way to furnish the amount needed in the diet.

Don't boil water in aluminum pans or kettles; this seriously reduces the existing fluorine content.

COPPER

Copper is used by the body to store iron and release it to form hemoglobin for red blood cells. The need for copper is particularly important in the early months of life, and if the mother's intake is sufficient, infants will be born with a store of copper. Human milk is a good source of copper; cow's milk is a poor one.

Since copper is widely distributed in foods, there should

presumably be no problem in meeting the U.S. RDA of 2 mg a day. However, there is some evidence, as described earlier, that we are not getting as much copper as we need. If, as the animal studies show, a deficiency in copper can lead to elevated levels of plasma cholesterol, good sense indicates that we should make sure to get an adequate supply of copper.

Copper occurs in most unprocessed foods. The richest sources are nuts, some shellfish, liver, kidney, raisins, and dried legumes.

CHROMIUM

Chromium, acting with insulin, is required for glucose utilization. A deficiency can produce a diabetes-like condition. Although not enough is known about the dietary role of chromium to set a recommended allowance, the Food and Nutrition Board says that studies indicate there may be marginal deficiencies, specifically among old people and pregnant women.

Good sources of chromium are most animal proteins (but not fish), whole grains, and brewer's yeast.

CHAPTER 9

Fiber

THERE IS, PERHAPS, no easier indicator to what has happened to the American diet than the latest nutritional buzzword, *fiber*. Back in the days when most food was unprocessed and unrefined and complex carbohydrates were the bulwark of our diet, fiber was called roughage and roughage was a natural component of the foods that everyone ate. As food processing grew into a multibillion-dollar industry, it created the environment for a flourishing business in laxatives.

Now that we have belatedly been made aware of the actual and possible consequences of the loss of fiber in our diet, the same food industry has rushed to help swing the pendulum the other way. Typically, the solution too often is another new product with another new additive. If there is anything more ludicrous than adding wood fiber to bread to replace the natural grain fiber lost in processing, it surely must be the addition of wood fiber to Kellogg's All-Bran, "a natural food-fiber cereal."

Do we need fiber? Do we need to get it from wood? The answer to the first question is yes, to the second, definitely not — it is not only ridiculous, it may cause constipation, the very condition it is supposed to prevent.

It is simpler to say where fiber is found than precisely what it is. Scientists are still not in complete agreement as to exactly what constitutes fiber, nor do they concur on how much is really needed and how lack of fiber relates to cancer and other diseases of the colon.

Fiber is present only in plant food in conjunction with the complex carbohydrates. There is no fiber in dairy products and none in meat, no matter how tough and fibrous it may seem. Fiber in plants is similar to the skeletal parts of the body: it provides structure to stems, leaves, fruit, and seeds. In grain the outside coat or bran layer is pure fiber. In general, fiber includes the skins and "woody" material in fruits, vegetables, and grains.

Although there are a number of different kinds of fiber in plants, they are usually lumped together as "dietary fiber." The fiber from wood, primarily lignum fiber, is generally described as "non-nutritive crude fiber."

In the body, fiber is the part of the plant that is not (or not much) absorbed. As it passes through the digestive system it absorbs water and remains bulky. The result is a stool that is soft and easy to pass and one that does not remain overlong in the intestine — in other words, just the opposite of the small, hard, constipated stool so typical of people in the Western world.

In modern times, the role of fiber was first brought to our attention as recently as the early 1970s by a medical practitioner in Africa. Dr. Dennis P. Burkitt, observing the rarity in natives of cancer of the colon and other diseases of the digestive tract, contrasted this with the high incidence of these same ailments in Western populations and attributed the difference to the fiber deficiency in our diet. Other studies have linked lack of fiber to heart disease, again on the basis of contrasting the incidence of heart disease in the West with its absence in populations that eat foods high in unrefined carbohydrates.

While the scientific answers aren't all in, the nutritional guidelines are clear. Fiber, once an important part of our diet, is just as important today. The question is how to restore it.

The best way is naturally, by increasing the consumption of complex carbohydrates, according to the Dietary Goals, all across the board — fruits, vegetables, whole grains, and legumes. Occasionally, for people unaccustomed to these foods, an increase in fiber may cause gas, but this is a temporary matter that will disappear as your intestines become adjusted to the more natural food.

When fruits and vegetables are frozen, some fiber is lost; when they are canned, the losses are more considerable. But the biggest loss in food processing takes place when flour is refined.

Although all natural, unprocessed carbohydrates contain fiber, some foods have more than others. As a guide, here are the best sources in each category:

Fruits: apples, bananas, berries, dried figs, oranges, pears, and raisins.

Vegetables: asparagus, beets, broccoli, corn, eggplant, green peas, all kinds of greens, lima beans, sweet potatoes, and summer squash.

Legumes: dried black-eyed, kidney, lima, navy, pinto beans, and soybeans; lentils and dried peas.

Grains and seeds: bran, bulgur, millet, oatmeal, rolled oats, sunflower seeds, and whole wheat.

CHAPTER 10

Additives

MORE THAN 1300 ADDITIVES are currently approved for
use as colors, flavors, preservatives, thickeners, and other
agents for controlling the physical properties of the food
we eat. They range from safe and necessary, to presently
necessary but not necessarily safe, to unsafe and unnecessary — with gradations along the way. Some of them are
there to give what food companies call "mouthfeel" to a
product that would otherwise taste like the test-tube conglomeration of chemicals it actually is.

The sheer numbers and pervasiveness of the substances
added to food, punctuated by periodic news that some
"safe" additive has belatedly been found to cause cancer —
ironically, "long-term usage" is actually one criterion for
calling an additive safe — have led to deep concern and considerable confusion among consumers. What can we do?
Who's to know which of a thousand chemicals in the
hundreds of food products in any supermarket are safe? And
is it a good idea, anyway, to introduce more and more new
substances, including some that don't occur in nature, into
our bodies?

For some of us, the answer is to choose only foods that
contain no additives at all, although "natural" foods may
contain sugar and salt, the two most overused and un-
healthy additives. At the other extreme, the cynical are
forced to conclude that "food is dangerous to your health,"
so you might as well stop worrying and eat everything. Con-

sidering the current selection of food products, both sides have a point; however, most of us would like an answer that lies somewhere between these two extremes. Without becoming paranoid over the possibility of eating any unidentifiable substance or obsessed with the need to memorize unpronounceable chemical names, we'd like to feel that what we eat is safe — and that we are not being forced to eat whatever a food manufacturer wants to give us.

If you observe the following guidelines (some of which are explained in detail later), you'll find that by taking just a few precautions you can avoid eating the most dubious additives and reduce the total amount in your food.

1. Wherever possible use fresh foods or processed foods that contain no additives.

2. Compare labels on different brands of the same food products. Among the additives that some manufacturers find necessary and others don't are the dubious antioxidants BHT and BHA and the flavor enhancer monosodium glutamate (no longer permitted in baby food but pretty ubiquitous elsewhere). Select the product with the fewest additives — with none at all if you can find it — and remember to include sugar and salt in that category.

3. Avoid foods that have artificial coloring.

4. Avoid foods that have sodium nitrate or sodium nitrite, especially bacon.

5. Don't eat food with saccharin except on doctor's orders.

6. Especially if you have children, invest $2.00 in a colorful poster called Chemical Cuisine and post it in the kitchen. The poster describes safe additives, ones to avoid, and ones to be cautious about. Although it is a handy reference for anyone, it's an excellent way to let children educate themselves — their favorite junk foods may be less appealing when they compare what's on the labels with the chart. The poster is available from the Center for Science in the Public Interest, 1755 S Street NW, Washington, DC 20009.

Most artificial colorings (about 95 percent of them) are synthetic chemicals derived from coal tar. Some are safer than others, but since the name of the dye does not appear on the label, you have no way of telling which coal-tar coloring is in the food. In the past, several of these dyes have been banned — Green #1, Violet #1, and Red #2. Although Orange B received FDA approval in 1966, after twelve years of making it, the manufacturer discovered that it contained a carcinogen and stopped producing it. According to the Center for Science in the Public Interest, some of these dyes are poorly tested, while others cause cancer in animals.

Beyond the question of safety, there are other good reasons to ban artificial dyes from your diet. These colorings are used primarily in junk food and foods of low nutritional value — candy, sodas, fruit drinks, packaged gelatin desserts, pastries, and even pet foods. A food with artificial coloring is almost always loaded with other additives, including sugar. By the single act of eliminating artificial coloring, you will automatically cut out a lot of sugar, salt, and other additives from your diet.

Although some additives to food are there for more or less beneficial reasons, there is absolutely no benefit to the consumer from these colorings. They do benefit the manufacturer, who puts them in because they make food look more attractive or even nutritious, so we are motivated to buy them. And of course they are perfectly right. How many people would buy a jar of colorless, tasteless chemicals called Tang and think it was a substitute for orange juice?

There are a few exceptions. One is beta carotene, a nutrient converted to vitamin A by the body. It is used to color butter, margarine, and certain other products. When it is used on foods that must contain a list of ingredients (butter and margarine don't have to) it is identified by name on the label.

Sodium Nitrate and Sodium Nitrite

These chemicals will be out of the food supply by 1982. Actually, they should have been banned in 1978, as soon as a government-sponsored study showed that they are carcinogenic in animals. However, Congress was asked to waive the law and allow a delay because while they can cause cancer, they can also prevent botulism. Consumer groups question the need for the delay on the grounds that safer preservatives are available and that manufacturers use nitrites as much for the pink color they impart to cured meats as for their qualities as a preservative.

Sodium nitrate and its derivative nitrite are used in 7 percent of the foods we eat including smoked fish, bacon, ham, sausage, corned beef, luncheon meats, and frankfurters. In the past they were used in baby foods, where admittedly they were intended as a coloring agent, not a preservative, since the jars were sterilized and sealed.

The biggest hazard of nitrites (aside from human errors when people have died after pouring it on food, mistaking it for salt or a meat tenderizer) is their ability to combine with other chemicals to form nitrosamines, which are highly carcinogenic. High heat, especially, turns nitrites into nitrosamines, which is why bacon is a food particularly to avoid. Bacon without nitrite is already on the market; so are frankfurters. Presumably, as the deadline approaches, safer preservatives will be found for all of these foods. (They will still be too fatty and generally too salty to be used regularly in the diet.)

Saccharin and Other Low-Calorie Sweeteners

In 1970, after years of repeated warnings by the National Academy of Sciences and other respected scientific groups, the FDA banned the artificial sweetener cyclamate on the grounds that it can cause cancer and birth defects. This sent the soft-drink manufacturers and other major users of artificial sweeteners back to saccharin, a substance that has been controversial since the early fifties, but which lacked the clear-cut proof of harm that finally brought down cyclamates.

By 1977, when the bad news about saccharin was in, the FDA proposed that it, too, be banned. This time an aroused public joined the manufacturers in demanding that saccharin be allowed. For diabetics the argument was that it was certainly safer than sugar. As of this writing, saccharin is still on the list of substances that may be added to foods, but it should definitely be avoided except on the advice of a doctor.

Mannitol is chemically similar to sugar, but because it is not quite as sweet and is also poorly absorbed by the body, it has about half the calories of sugar and is far less likely to cause cavities in teeth. Mannitol is frequently used in low-calorie foods and in sugarless chewing gum. It has been used for centuries as a natural sweetener and is considered perfectly safe. Look for it instead of saccharin on the label of low-calorie foods.

BHA and BHT

Although BHA and BHT are on the FDA list of GRAS (generally regarded as safe) substances, they are also generally regarded, even by the FDA, as being poorly tested. In 1976, the FDA recommended that they be removed until further studies could determine their safety, but nothing has been done. BHA is presumed to be somewhat better than BHT. These additives are widely used in cereals, convenience foods, potato chips, chewing gum, and bakery products, to stabilize fats and oils and prolong shelf life. Safer substances are usually available.

Added Nutrients

Although some additives like the emulsifier lecithin, the artificial coloring carotene, and the antioxidant alpha tocopherol (vitamin E) are indeed nutrients, they are added to food for reasons other than their nutritional qualities. When vitamins and minerals are added to food *specifically* for reasons of nutrition, those foods are called fortified or enriched.

If a food is described as *fortified*, it means that nutrients not originally in the food (or in it in insignificant amounts) are added. An example of sensible fortification is milk, which is fortified with vitamins A and D. Milk is rich in protein and calcium and obviously important for growing children. However, calcium needs the presence of vitamin D to be absorbed in the body, and vitamin D is not plentiful in food. Adding it to milk ensures that we get both needed calcium and vitamin D. The case for adding vitamin A is not quite so clear; however, it is reasonable enough, since vitamin A needs vitamin D to be properly used.

When milk is fortified, it is a case of making a nutritious food better. When imitation fruit drinks and sugary cereals are fortified, it's strictly a sales pitch to convince parents that the food is good for the kids. Adding vitamins doesn't reduce the amount of sugar and additives; bad food is still bad food. A new entry into the fortified junk food game is a chocolate candy "nutrition bar," a synthetic conglomeration of "essential" vitamins and minerals — and a lot of nonessential additives. The chemical flavor of this candy makes one long for the honest taste and guilt of a plain old chocolate bar.

Food is described as *enriched* when nutrients that have been removed in the processing are later replaced. The reason some people seem to save their worst ire for enriched foods is that the term is basically a fraud. If you remove something and then replace it, that isn't enrichment. More serious, though, is the fact that only *some* of the nutrients lost are replaced. So, although foods that are enriched are better than they would be were they not enriched, they aren't as good as the original before anything was removed or replaced. The obvious example is enriched white flour, which is better than unenriched flour but not as good as the whole wheat flour from which it was made.

There is nothing inherently wrong with enrichment and fortification of foods. What is wrong is confusing enriched sugar-coated breakfast cereals or fortified candy nutrition bars with real food. A potential threat, however, is the unknown amount of "good" additives we may accumulate as the number of enriched and fortified foods we consume grows constantly larger.

Part II

Selecting, Storing, and Preparing Foods: Making the Goals a Reality

CHAPTER 11

Vegetables

VEGETABLES, AS EVERYBODY KNOWS, are good for you, but that fact alone isn't very helpful. You need information about which ones to choose and how to conserve their food value when you get them home. All parts of the varied plants we eat as vegetables offer vitamins and minerals, from A, B, and C through Z for zinc. Some few vegetables are high in practically all nutrients, others are less so. Should you then serve broccoli stems and leaves four times a week and collard greens the remaining three, thus cornering the nutrition market? Hardly. Eating is for enjoyment, and variety is a necessary seasoning. Besides, a wide selection is the first step toward a total nutritional coverage.

Consider the vegetables you eat now and, on your next trip to the store, see what's offered. Try chard or beet tops or broccoli rabe instead of relying on spinach as the only leafy green in your repertoire. If corn, string beans, peas, and carrots are the outer limits of your vegetable world, it's going to take a certain firmness to broaden out. Think of it as consciousness-raising and remember it's all habit. The collard greens one person scorns are a southerner's delight.

Because the vitamins in vegetables are comparatively unstable, they begin to dwindle when they leave the earth. This means we need to know ways to ensure getting the maximum food value from what we've bought.

Most of us have some personal formula by which we decide which vegetables to eat fresh, which frozen, and which canned — fresh carrots, frozen peas, and canned beets, for example. To a degree, these choices make sense: fresh salad greens, naturally; frozen lima beans because fresh ones aren't available; and canned corn occasionally because it is so convenient. Where patterns are based on habit, however, this might be a good time to reassess them, taking into consideration nutrition, taste, convenience, and cost.

Although conventional wisdom holds fresh vegetables to be more nutritious than their processed counterparts, this may not be true in all places at all times. In season, locally grown produce (if fresh) is always the best nutritional buy. At other times of year, fresh produce shipped across the country may undergo considerable nutrient depletion by the time it gets to market. Under those circumstances, frozen vegetables, which are usually processed hours after harvesting, probably retain more vitamins than the "fresh" ones, though they *may* not taste as good. Fresh broccoli, carrots, cauliflower, zucchini, and many others may have better consistency and taste even out of season than their frozen counterparts. Although vegetables are also canned shortly after harvesting, there is greater loss of most nutrients in canning than in freezing.

Fresh Vegetables

Since few supermarkets or food cooperatives receive daily shipments of perishable foods, ask the clerk in the produce department when your store gets its deliveries. If the schedule is Monday and Friday, try not to buy food like string beans on Thursday evening because chances are you'll find only limp leftovers. A few days more or less may not seem significant in light of the total time spent in transcontinental shipment, but vegetables undergo more abuse in the store than in refrigerator trucks or cold warehouses.

Select crisp, firm, unwilted vegetables with good color. Look over the whole plant, even if you actually use just a part of it, because bruised tissue indicates some loss of vitamin C.

Frozen Vegetables

Frozen food should be considered perishable and carefully examined before purchase; if it has been defrosted and refrozen, it suffers in both nutrition and taste. Reject any package that has visible signs of leakage or accumulated "snow." Frozen packages should be perfectly shaped; if they are rounded on one side or misshapen in any way, that is a sure sign that they defrosted somewhere in transit. Vegetables in plastic bags should be frozen hard but loose; a solid frozen block is an indication of melting and refreezing.

Frozen vegetables are truly one of the great convenience foods, but the processors have not seen fit to let a good product stand on its merits. There is more money to be made by immersing a smaller quantity of vegetables in a fattening sauce, especially when the so-called gourmet dish has a higher price tag. These days, frozen-food shelves seem to have more vegetables in sauce than plain ones.

On the other hand, bags of mixed frozen vegetables can be a convenience for use in soups and stews or to provide variety as a side dish. When you buy mixed vegetables, you should balance taste against convenience, since one bag may contain both vegetables that freeze well and those that have a mealy or watery consistency when frozen.

Canned Vegetables

These are generally somewhat lower in nutrients than either fresh or frozen produce. They are always higher in salt and lower in fiber. (If sodium is a problem, buy low-salt rather than regular canned goods.) So, although canned vegetables lose out on the basis of nutrition, they are often a good choice for convenience, cost, and availability. Beets, to take one food, are never frozen and not always to be found fresh, so if you want to eat them, the only choice is canned. As for canned tomatoes, especially the plum variety for sauces, stews, and soups, who would want to cook without them?

Canned foods are not, of course, perishable, but there may be nutrient loss if you keep cans for a long time at a warm temperature. Stored at 80°F, canned vegetables can lose up to one-quarter of their vitamin C and thiamin. Store canned staples that you keep around for a long time at 65°F.

To get your money's worth from canned vegetables, save the liquids for soup or stock — the water-soluble vitamins belong to you. Naturally, this goes for the water you use to cook fresh or frozen vegetables too. Keep a jar in the refrigerator or freezer and add the cooking liquid to what you have on hand.

Finally, remember the Dietary Goal for salt, and don't add more salt to the sodium already in the canned vegetables.

Vitamins and Minerals

Selection, storage, washing, and cooking all affect the amount of nutrients you get from vegetables. In leafy greens or yellow vegetables, the deeper the color, the more vitamin A the vegetable has. Since the B complex vitamins as well as vitamin C, an important nutrient in many vegetables, are all water-soluble, don't clean vegetables by letting them soak in water. Wash them, preferably just before using, as briefly as possible to remove the dirt. Tight heads of lettuce or cabbage need rinsing only on the outside. Even notoriously sandy foods like spinach or asparagus can be cleaned of dirt by swooshing them through a few changes of water rather than letting them soak away their vitamins. Except where noted later in this chapter, store vegetables in the refrigerator, either in the hydrator or in a loose plastic bag with air holes. Some vitamins will be lost even in the refrigerator so, to the extent that your schedule allows, buy fresh produce in small quantities. Use opened cans or frozen vegetables right away, and don't let any vegetables stand around exposed to light, heat, or air for any length of time. Keep them covered and refrigerated until you are ready to use them, and do the same with leftovers.

Water-soluble vitamins suffer the most extensive loss in cooking. To minimize this, cook vegetables for the shortest possible time in the smallest amount of water, and save the cooking liquid for stock. To get rid of the air in the water, bring it to a boil before adding the vegetable. Even better, invest in an inexpensive steamer that fits right into your regular pots, and steam the vegetables, again briefly. Or stir-fry them in a wok until just crisp, using a very small amount of polyunsaturated oil.

Some people advocate pressure cookers to save vitamins, but we're not among them. True, cooking time is shortened, but the vitamin-saving effect is not appreciable, since vegetables rarely require long cooking anyway. The real trouble is that it is almost impossible, we find, to control the degree of doneness of pressure-cooked food. Vegetables are almost invariably overcooked, while the starch in legumes tends to clog the petcock.

For foods that require lengthy cooking in a minimum amount of water, a heavy aluminum, steel, or enamel-coated pot is a good investment. A heavy iron pot is particularly useful since it becomes a source of iron in your diet. (Don't use it for cooking foods that are important sources of vitamin C.) Whatever your choice of pan, always cook vegetables covered, and *don't* use sodium bicarbonate, which destroys thiamin and vitamin C.

If vegetables have never been a favorite food, it may be that you've always had them overcooked. Considering how easy it is to cook vegetables, it is remarkable how rarely they are cooked correctly. There's a gastronomic light year of difference between soft, limp vegetables and the same food cooked until just barely tender. The latter are sweet instead of bitter, with a fresh fragrance and better, brighter color.

Go a step further and eat vegetables raw whenever you can. There are very few vegetables, either cooked or raw, that don't enhance a salad. Some, like string beans or broccoli, are improved if they are briefly blanched before they are used in salad. Leftover cooked vegetables are almost always better cold in salad than reheated, but if you do reheat vegetables, remember that you are just reheating them, not recooking them.

There are some delightful vegetables — among them cucumber, celery, and eggplant — that are not listed in this chapter because they're not very high in nutrients, though of course we use them, usually in combination with others. Celery and cucumber are great snacks, are easy to handle, and offer some bulk. Others are extravagances, such as asparagus and artichokes, which we eat occasionally without really thinking of their nutrients, just reveling in their taste.

Avocado

Botanically, the avocado, like the tomato, is a fruit, but since salad is its most typical environment, we put the avocado in this chapter. One of the few vegetable sources of niacin, and with a good amount of vitamin C and potassium, avocados are, unlike most vegetables, high in fat and rich in calories. They are ripe when they give under gentle pressure, but the hard ones will ripen perfectly at room temperature — it's just a matter of planning ahead if you are going to use them for a special dinner. Some have smooth skins, others are darker and rougher, but all varieties are delicious. If you use just half of the avocado, leave the pit in the other half, squeeze some lemon or lime juice on the exposed flesh, and wrap it tightly in plastic wrap — and keep it in the refrigerator, of course.

Beets

The most nutritious part of the beet is not the tuber but the tops, which are an excellent source of vitamin A when they are fresh. If you are lucky enough to find beets with their tops on, look for tubers of the same size (so they will cook in the same amount of time) and tops that are crisp and whole, not leathery and bug-nibbled. The young leaves are excellent in salad; cook the older ones as you would any other leafy green. Use the perishable tops the day you buy them; store the tubers unwashed in a plastic bag in the hydrator.

Broccoli

In a famous old *New Yorker* cartoon, a mother urges her little girl to "Eat your broccoli, darling." The child replies, "I say it's spinach and I say the hell with it." It's a toss-up which of these two vegetables is the more nutritious, but only dreadfully overcooked broccoli could be mistaken for spinach.

Broccoli is extremely high in vitamins A and C, and since all parts of the plant are good, look for close flower heads with tight small buds, firm stalks, and crisp leaves. The greener the color, the more nutrients. The leaves, which most people strip off, have the most vitamin A; the stalks are tender and delicious if you simply pare off the outside skin. Broccoli takes very well to cooking in a steamer. Cut up the bottom stalks and put the pieces in first; then stand up the rest of the stalks with the flower heads upright. Cook broccoli until it is just barely tender, and if the rest of the dinner isn't quite ready, take the broccoli out of the pot or it will overcook and also lose its bright green color. Cold broccoli, cooked this way, is excellent in a mixed salad.

Brussels Sprouts

Like its relatives, this tiny member of the cabbage family is a good source of vitamin C. Select tight, green heads; loose and yellowing leaves are a sign of age. More than anything else, overcooked Brussels sprouts seem to be responsible for the bad reputation of English cooking. They *are* dreadful that way, but when cooked until just crisp and tender, they are delicate and delicious. If you cut a cross slash in the stem end of the sprout, the heart and the leaves will cook through in the same length of time. Keep it short.

Cabbage

This is an excellent vegetable to keep on hand for salads as well as for cooking, since it suffers less nutrient loss in storage than most other vegetables. Green cabbage has somewhat more vitamin C than the red variety, but both are good sources of vitamins, minerals, and fiber. Use the outside leaves unless they're limp and broken, and cut them smaller.

Carrots

This is another vegetable that keeps its nutrients well when stored in the hydrator. Carrots, as their bright orange color indicates, are a good source of vitamin A among other nutrients. The orange mature carrot has several times as much A as the paler young ones, but both have so much that it doesn't really matter. Because carrots are sweet, they make a good raw snack. Keep them accessible.

Carrots retain their sweet taste if cooked just barely firm. At the soft stage they are overcooked.

Cauliflower

Cauliflower is a very good source of vitamin C, especially raw. Look for a creamy white head with crisp green leaves, and pass up cauliflower that is bruised and spotty. Cauliflower doesn't keep well, so use it up quickly. Raw flowerets are good in salad or with a dip.

Green Peas

Niacin, magnesium, and vitamin C are the most important nutrients in green peas. When your market has fresh peas, look for crisp, full, but not oversized pods. The color should indeed be pea green, not yellowish. Frozen peas are a better buy than average, poor quality, fresh ones. Avoid canned peas because of the high sodium and low potassium content.

Lettuce

If iceberg lettuce is an ingrained habit, try to nudge it a bit. The other lettuces, romaine and the loose-leaf varieties, have more nutrients and much more taste. If you do buy iceberg, don't throw away the tougher outside leaves with all their vitamin A. Shred them up and mix them in with the more tender greens or add them to soups at the last minute. Store lettuce in the hydrator.

Greens

These include spinach, kale, chard, collards, or any other green that might appear in your market. Lately broccoli rabe — the leaves and small flowerets of the plant — are being sold separately as greens in many stores. In all these, look for good color, crispness, a fresh quality, and no little holes that tell the insects have been there first. Between pre-washed bagged and loose unwashed spinach, make the judgment according to how fresh the loose appears to be and how rushed you are.

In some vegetables the unfamiliar parts are more nutritious, such as the stalks and stems of broccoli; but in spinach, kale, and collard greens the leaves have more nutrients than the stems or the midribs, so remember to strip the more tender parts away from the older stalks when you are preparing them for cooking.

Mushrooms

What makes mushrooms so good is not their inherent nutritional value, which is not outstanding, but their ability to enhance the taste of other foods, whether used raw in salads or cooked in sauces. Loose mushrooms, if your store still carries them, are usually more expensive than the ones that come in packages. But look at the label on the package; if you see sodium bisulphite in fine print, a preservative has been used. Although the mushrooms *look* fresh, they have been held for a much longer time than really fresh mushrooms, and the quality is inferior. Another form of packaged mushroom is golden in color. These are usually very dirty and, unlike the white ones, have to be soaked and scrubbed to get clean. As with so many other foods, your

choice of what is available is determined by the food industry or your supermarket.

Onions

Dear to the heart of every cook, onions are also a pretty
good source of vitamin C and potassium. Globe onions —
yellow, white, red, Bermuda, and Spanish — should be firm
and dry when you buy them. If they come in a mesh bag,
inspect and poke each one to be sure they aren't soft or
sprouted; there always seems to be a bad onion in the bag.
Globe onions keep best at about 55°F. If possible, store only
a few loose onions in your warm kitchen (not in the refrigerator) and keep the rest in a cooler closet. Scallions or green
onions should be stored in the refrigerator in a plastic bag
with air space or in the hydrator.

Sweet Peppers

Extremely high in vitamin C, a pretty good source of A
and some minerals, and delicious to boot, green peppers are
too good to be used merely as a decorative addition to a
salad plate. The big news is that *red* sweet peppers (the
green ones ripen into red) are almost twice as high in vitamin C and offer more than ten times the amount of vitamin A. And a strip of red sweet pepper is so full of natural
sugar it can serve as a snack substitute for candy. Buy firm
and unwrinkled peppers with no soft spots.

Potatoes

Although they're overrated on the calorie scale and under-
rated as a nutritious food, everybody likes the taste of potatoes. Unfortunately, they are most popular in their least nutritious, most caloric forms. Next time the waitress asks,
"Baked or French fried?" you might want to think back to
the table on the next page.

Naturally, if you put butter on the baked potato, you will
increase the number of calories and the fat. However, in pro-

POTATO	CALO-RIES	PRO-TEIN (G)	FAT (G)	IRON (MG)	THIA-MIN (MG)	RIBO-FLAVIN (MG)	NIA-CIN (MG)	VITA-MIN C (MG)
1 Baked	145	4.2	0.2	1.1	.15	.07	2.7	31
10 French fries (frozen, heated)	172	2.8	6.6	1.4	.11	.02	2.0	16
10 Chips	114	1.1	8.0	0.4	.04	.01	1.0	3

tein and vitamins, the baked potato is still a far more nutritious food than either the French fries or the potato chips.

Like all vegetables potatoes contain the most nutrients when they're fresh, but this is a considerably longer period than in the case of leafy greens. However, it makes sense to choose the freshest variety.

All purpose: In the northeastern and central states the big suppliers are Maine and Long Island. The staple varieties begin to be harvested at the end of August and continue until freezing weather. This means that winter and spring potatoes coming to market from these sources will have been stored.

Russets: These are most often from Idaho, long and oval in shape, and are harvested slightly later than the all-purpose kind. Winter and spring potatoes come from storage. Their low water content makes russets very good bakers.

"New" potatoes appear in early spring from the warm growing regions of the South and West. The Floridas are usually red-skinned and small; the Californias are light tan, all sizes, and lovely for cooking in their skin.

All potatoes should have good color for their variety, which means no green. Select dry potatoes; damp ones will be rotten.

Summer Squash

The summer squashes, including zucchini, are good sources of vitamin C, with fair amounts of vitamin A and minerals. Since this is a vegetable you can eat raw or cooked, get the maximum nutrients by at least occasionally having these raw. Eat them plain, cut in strips. With a curried yogurt dip they're terrific. Look for firmness, small size, and good shape with no dwindled-down soft ends.

Winter Squash

Somewhat less known in some parts of the country, the various winter squashes have more vitamin A and minerals, including iron, than summer squash. Their season is primarily the fall and winter months. The following varieties are those you'll be likely to find in the store.

Hubbard, the largest, is a grayish blue, kind of whale-shaped vegetable, sometimes bumpy of skin. The flesh is yellow. Often Hubbard is sold in pieces, which is useful if you want to sample it to see if you like the taste, but it's really not wise to buy it in this form.

Butternut has a long neck and a full body and is a muted golden yellow in color, both in skin and flesh.

Acorn is smaller than butternut, is oval and ridged, and usually deep green in color with splashes of yellowish orange. The flesh is yellow, sometimes with an orange cast.

Buttercup is the best tasting winter squash, though hard to find. It is round with straight, up-and-down sides and a little turban on top. Like acorn, it is deep green with yellow patches. The flesh, however, is deep orange with a delicious texture and taste.

String Beans

Although they are not outstanding vegetables nutritionally — except insofar as all fresh vegetables are good sources of fiber — string beans are generally a favorite. Select young beans with good color, and conserve the vitamin C by cooking them briefly. Use fresh beans immediately; save leftover cold beans for salads for the next day.

Tomatoes

To be able to eat fresh fruits and vegetables in the middle of winter is truly one of the miracles of modern food production. The remarkable thing about most out-of-season produce is how closely it approximates garden-picked food. One sorry exception is the tomato, which under normal circumstances cannot stand either rough handling or long transit. Yet the mealy, tasteless object that passes for a tomato in the market today is not an ordinary tomato that suffered in shipping, but a specially engineered product designed for mass production and mass consumption under the harshest of conditions. Its uniform size, perfectly round shape, and tough skin were bred into it by plant geneticists whose goal was to develop a tomato that could be picked by machine. So far so good, but even a perfectly round tomato with a rugged skin won't ship well if the inside is sweet and juicy. To minimize losses (and maximize profits), commercial tomatoes are picked when they are green and hard. Along the way they do turn red (with an assist from ethylene gas), but that is about all they have in common with a ripe tomato. Among the losses is much of the tomato's chief nutrient, vitamin C.

In the past, we could at least count on vine-ripened tomatoes in the summer months. With the success of the commercial tomato, however, tomatoes are picked green even during peak harvest times. In summer, of course, you can get real tomatoes, if not from your garden, from a farm stand. If they aren't fully ripe when you get them, stand them stem side up in a moderately warm room out of the sun. When they are ripe, put them in the refrigerator. Unfortunately, this method doesn't work well with the commercial tomatoes; they just get mealier and more watery, so put them right in the refrigerator and make the best of it. Or save your money and add color to salads with cheaper, tastier, more nutritious alternatives such as sweet red peppers, red cabbage, and radishes. Canned stewed tomatoes make a good hot vegetable and taste more like tomatoes than the ersatz fresh thing.

Turnips

Though not everybody's favorite, turnips have hidden virtues: a goodly amount of vitamin C and some thiamin. The green part of the plant has the most nutrients, including vitamin A. In most commercial markets, turnips are sold with a paraffin dip as a preservative, which should be peeled off before cooking. Turnip greens are sold separately, but not in all parts of the country. South of the Mason-Dixon line they are universally available.

Watercress

Crisp, pungent watercress, an excellent addition to salads for texture and taste, is also a superior source of vitamin A, as one might expect from the deep green color. Never buy limp watercress that the clerk assures you will perk up when you soak it. It will, indeed, but the nutrients are gone forever. Store watercress in a plastic bag or stand it up like a bunch of flowers in a glass of water — in the refrigerator, of course.

Yams or Sweet Potatoes

These delicious tubers are excellent sources of nutrients — as long as they're prepared without sugary additions. A single baked sweet potato has half the amount of vitamin C needed for a day and twice the amount of A.

Though neither is technically a yam (which is a similar looking vegetable popular in the West Indies) two types are sold commercially. The one known as a yam has a soft, moist texture when cooked, with very sweet orange to orange-red flesh. The skin may be orange, pink, or copper-red.

The second type has firm, dry, and mealy flesh when cooked, and lighter skin. Canned sweet potatoes are often of this variety, which adds to their uninteresting taste.

Unlike white potatoes, yams don't store well. Buy dry, firm vegetables, and only enough for a meal or two.

Herbs and Spices

If you're confused about the difference between herbs and spices, it's a rather precious one. Herbs are the leaves and flowers of certain plants and are used preferably fresh, but also dried and frozen. Tarragon, dill, basil, and oregano are examples, as well as the most common herb, parsley.

Spices can be leaves or flowers, but are generally berries or the roots and bark of shrubs or small trees. Their form varies widely: ginger, for instance, can be used fresh or dry, whole or ground, sugared or preserved. Spices conjure up the wide world, from Madagascar cloves to Turkish bay leaves to Indian turmeric. In earlier days their great importance was in preserving, not masking bad-tasting food as is sometimes said.

In buying herbs and spices, think small. If your only source is the supermarket, pick the smallest amounts sold, and where there are two brands offered, the more expensive jar is not necessarily the best buy if it's been sitting on the shelf for a year. The cheaper tin may be preferable. If, however, there's a good turnover and the shelves are restocked often, the glass jarred products are often superior. If you have access to a proper spice store, where you can select and weigh your purchases, bring them home and transfer them to the smallest jars you can find. Be sure the tops are screwed on tight and mark the date of purchase on each one. Store them away from heat — not over the stove. Replenish ground or crushed leaves every six to nine months. Whole berries such as pepper and allspice, or whole bay leaf, cloves, and cinnamon bark can be held longer.

The following are useful herbs for a variety of dishes:

Parsley

Fresh parsley is usually found in its curled variety, though the straight, or Italian, is frequently available, sometimes with its root intact. (This is a good addition to soup.) Don't think of parsley as only a decorative addition to a platter: it is rich in vitamins A and C and iron. Since it is long lasting in the hydrator, it's hard to think why one would want the dusty, tasteless stuff sold as dried parsley.

Basil

Sweet basil is the leaf of a rather attractive plant, easy to grow indoors or out. Use it in any cooked dish that includes tomato, but it comes into its glory minced fresh on a raw tomato and onion salad. If you grow a few plants you'll have enough to freeze or dry. Both are simple to do. Cut the leaves in the morning when they are good-sized but flowers have not yet appeared on the plant. Rinse well and spread them out to dry off. Discard the less-than-perfect leaves. For drying, tie a bunch together in some dry, warm, clean place.

To freeze basil, cut the stems short and place the clean leaves in a plastic bag, seal, and place in the freezer. The leaves can be broken off when needed in cooking.

Oregano

We find this to be an overworked herb that should be limited to some dishes cooked Mediterranean style. Oregano and salads are a poor combination in our mind, and it doesn't go well with vegetables, or at least not in the quantities in which it is often found. Buy it in leaf, not powdered, form.

Marjoram

This is an optional but handy herb, somewhat similar to oregano but used more discriminately by most of us. Again, buy the leaves, not the powder.

Sage

Sage is an old American favorite, especially in stuffings. A little goes a long way. Use it in dishes that have a strength of their own, such as stews or soups, and not for anything very subtle.

Tarragon

This lovely, strong, rather sweet herb is much better when used fresh. A small sprig in the cavity of a roasting chicken gloriously perfumes the bird. Its use in vinegar is well known. If you have access to tarragon, immerse a small sprig in a bottle of wine vinegar for a few days. We don't recommend its being held in the vinegar indefinitely.

Thyme

There are many varieties of thyme, and if you have a garden you should try lemon and common thyme. For a pot indoors French thyme is good, since it grows more upright than the sprawly kinds. If you buy it in the store, get the dried leaves, not powder, and use it sparingly.

CHAPTER 12

Fruits

No one really has to make a case for fruits. Full of vitamins and minerals, they taste delicious and require less preparation than almost any other kind of food. Fruits play an especially important role in the protective nutrition of the Dietary Goals, since they are the most nutritious low-calorie food that is also satisfyingly sweet. The foods that fruits replace for desserts or snacks are the very ones often loaded with sugar, fats, and additives. Even their seasonal availability is a plus for fruits, since those we can eat for only a month or two are all the more a treat. Fortunately, though, there is a good variety at all seasons of the year.

Although a bowl of fresh fruit is a pleasant invitation to healthy snacking (to say nothing of a nice decorative touch), remember that unrefrigerated fruit loses vitamins. Once fruit has ripened, leave just a few pieces out and replenish the bowl from the refrigerator.

Many fruits don't freeze well, and unless you need something like frozen raspberries for a special dessert sauce, it's best to wait until the fresh fruit is available. While canned fruits are a marvelous convenience, the vitamins and fiber that are lost in processing are replaced tenfold by sugar. At least, try to buy canned fruit processed in light syrup or, better yet, in its own juice. Pineapple comes in its own juice and certainly needs no sugar, and some dietetic fruits are now canned in the juice of white grapes instead of sweetened with artificial sweeteners.

When it comes to fruits, some dieters have mysteriously been advised to avoid watermelon, cherries, and grapes on the grounds that these are high in calories. This is quite untrue; though cherries and grapes don't offer the most nutrients among fruits, all three have negligible calories when eaten in normal amounts. We compared the calories per pound of fruit, omitting oranges and grapefruit because our source, the Department of Agriculture Handbook #456, *Nutritive Value of American Foods*, does not compute these foods by the pound.

Watermelon	118	Calories per pound
Cantaloupe	136	
Peaches	141	
Honeydew melon	150	
Strawberries	168	
Grapes	207	
Pineapple	236	
Apples	263	
Cherries	318	
Bananas	386	

Apples

Perhaps the reason one of these a day was supposed to keep the doctor away is because raw apples are an excellent source of fiber, particularly the skin and the area just under it. These days, if you eat the skin of any apple, be sure to wash it first. If the apple resembles a piece of waxed fruit, it probably *was* waxed, and in that case, peel off the skin and discard it.

While apples are not a great source of vitamins compared to some other fruits, they do have valuable trace minerals in addition to the fiber. One of the least temperamental of fruits, apples are available all year long. The peak season for American apples is fall, when both taste and nutrition are at their best, but commercially "cooled" apples are a good buy at any time of year. The relatively new Granny Smith apples that come from Australia, with its topsy-turvy seasons, are an excellent choice for spring and summer.

Different parts of the country have their own favorites, but nationally Red Delicious, McIntosh, and Golden Delicious are the varieties of choice. Try a Macoun for an excellent crisp red apple or, if you have the opportunity, sample some of the older varieties, such as the Northern Spy, which are no longer widely sold commercially.

Cooked or canned apples are pleasant but have little to offer nutritionally.

Apricots

Undoubtedly, the *real* forbidden fruit on the tree in the Garden of Eden was the golden-cheeked apricot, apple enthusiasts notwithstanding. Apricots are widely available in many forms and are excellent sources of vitamin A when fresh, canned, or dried.

Commercially grown largely on the West Coast, fresh apricots are shipped fairly hard and are occasionally lacking in top flavor. Look for good-sized juicy ones.

Canned apricots are sometimes sold water packed, without additional sweetness of any kind. Usually, however, they're in a heavy syrup, in which case drain this and use it in making a gelatin of your own flavor. If you're serving the apricots in a liquid, stir together a little orange juice and a tablespoon or two of the canned apricot liquid. A tablespoon of a fruit liqueur is a delicious option.

Dried apricots are a concentrated source of iron as well as vitamin A, with only the unconscionably high current prices on the minus side. If you're worried about calories, ten medium dried apricots contain only 91 calories.

Bananas

Although they are slightly more caloric than other fruits, bananas are also more filling and therefore a good choice when you are hungry. On the basis of nutrition, cost, and year-round availability, bananas are one of our most valuable fruits. Moreover, unlike some other fruits that are to be found all year, the quality is generally high. The only trick is to eat them when they are exactly ripe, which is when the skin is yellow and shows some brown spots. You can buy bananas even when they are green; they'll ripen perfectly in the house at room temperature. If it looks as if they will become overripe before you are ready to use them up, store them in the refrigerator. The skins will blacken but the flesh will be just right. Use refrigerated bananas immediately after taking them out.

Cherries

Sweet cherries are, for fruit, comparatively low in nutrients, though they have a fair amount of vitamin A. Buy them firm and deep-colored. The bright red cherries are tart, and since the point of eating them is their sweet taste, avoid the lighter-colored ones.

Canned sour cherries are excellent sources of vitamin A and some C. However, this has to be balanced against the very large amount of sugar one needs to add to make them palatable.

Citrus Fruits

Oranges

The most popular fruit in America is the orange, consumed in largest part in the convenient form of reconstituted frozen juice. While orange juice is certainly nutritious, only the whole orange, with its valuable pulp, contains fiber.

The main orange-growing areas offer fresh oranges throughout most of the year; only in summer are you likely to find less-than-perfect fruit. California and the western states have two major oranges, the winter navel, the best of all eating oranges and the one with the highest proportion of vitamin C, and the summer Valencia. Florida's several varieties come to market from about October to late spring. Although they have slightly less vitamin C than the California varieties — comparing numbers here is nitpicking — *all* oranges are excellent sources of this vitamin as well as potassium and other minerals.

To get the most for your money, look for heavy oranges with thin skins. Navels are thick-skinned by nature, but even here you can usually select ones that appear thinner-skinned than others. The color of the orange is of no consequence; unlike most fruits, a slight greenish color doesn't indicate unripeness but merely that the nights were warm in the growing season. California oranges are not artificially colored; *some* Florida oranges may still be colored, but the color doesn't penetrate through the skin.

Store oranges and all citrus fruits in the refrigerator. They'll keep as long as six to eight weeks in the unlikely event that you don't use them up a lot sooner.

ORANGE JUICE: FROZEN JUICE VERSUS FROZEN JUICE DRINKS

Since all frozen concentrates have to be defrosted in exactly the same way, there must be a reason why someone would buy a frozen "orange breakfast beverage" or an "imitation orange juice" over the real thing, frozen orange juice concentrate. In truth, as a comparison shopping trip to the supermarket shows, there is no reason to buy the substitute and every reason why we shouldn't.

On one day, in one store, a 12-ounce container of any of several brands of frozen orange juice cost $1.13. All of them contained frozen concentrated orange juice, period.

A 12-ounce container of the "orange breakfast beverage," Birds Eye Orange Plus, cost a penny less, $1.12. Described as containing 30 percent orange juice, its primary ingredient was water (this is in addition to the water you add in mixing). The other pluses were two kinds of sugar, a mouthful of assorted additives including artificial color, artificial flavor, the synthetic preservative BHA, a bunch of vitamins, and "orange pulp." So, for the penny saved, you lose two-thirds of the orange juice and gain frozen water, sugar, and additives.

On the other hand, at 63 cents, 12 ounces of Birds Eye Awake did seem to be an economy — but only if it were possible to compare this "imitation orange juice" with real orange juice, or even Orange Plus. The label on Awake states that it contains no juice at all. In order of predominance, its major ingredients are sugar syrup, water, corn syrup (another form of sugar), and orange pulp. For the rest, it's a similar collection of additives and vitamins and so imitation that even vitamin C is added. Considering the cost of frozen water and chemicals, even the cheapest of these three drinks is a very poor buy compared to orange juice.

Grapefruits

Grapefruits are best from fall through spring — the summer ones are either dried out leftovers or the prematurely harvested new crop. Pink grapefruit is higher in vitamin A than the white Marsh variety. It's also considerably sweeter and never needs additional sugar, a point to keep in mind for people who automatically sugar their grapefruit.

Grapefruits are not quite as high in vitamin C as are oranges, but they are still one of the best sources of that vitamin. And they are lower in calories.

Other Citrus Fruits

Look for the thinnest-skinned lemons you can find, since the juice is what you want to spend your money on. A smooth skin usually indicates a juicy lemon. Limes are almost always thin-skinned and can be used interchangeably with lemons, according to whichever is better in quality and price. Tangerines have a short growing season and come to market between Thanksgiving and the middle of January. Tangelos, Murcotts, and Temple oranges are available through spring. The skin of the tangerine and its relatives will stand away from the flesh somewhat, but too much space between pulp and skin is an indication of dryness.

Dried Fruits

The intense sweetness and high mineral content of dried fruits make them one of the best substitutes for empty-calorie snacks. There are a couple of drawbacks: dried fruits have concentrated their sugar and are sticky, which makes them both comparatively caloric and caries-causing. Although it is far better for children to snack on raisins or dates than Twinkies or Chuckles, the natural sugar will stick to their teeth just as much as the processed sugar will.

When fruit is sun-dried it darkens. Light-colored dried fruits, particularly apricots and golden raisins, are treated with sulfur dioxide (which has been in use for more than a hundred years) or potassium sorbate to maintain their color. These preservatives, which are considered acceptable, also help retain moisture. If you buy packaged dried fruits, with or without an added preservative, purchase it from a store that has a high turnover to be sure it isn't stale or buggy. Store the fruit covered in the refrigerator.

Grapes

Though grapes are among the lowest in nutrients of all fruits, they're a far better snack than one of the usual junk foods. Today's grapes have considerably more water in them as a result of agricultural tinkering, which hasn't added to their flavor or firmness.

All the varieties are about the same in food value.

Melons

We've never known anyone who didn't like melons, yet our national consumption of melons is only half what it was in the early 1900s. The decline is probably related to the fact that melons are rarely, if ever, found in cans, frozen packages, or as juice. And since we aren't likely to equate melons with high nutrition, their often high price makes them seem like a luxury fruit.

Surprisingly, of all the fruits we eat, melons are the most

loaded with vitamins and minerals, particularly vitamins A and C, potassium, and iron. In his *Nutrition Scoreboard,* Dr. Michael Jacobson of the Center for Science in the Public Interest ranks fresh fruits on the basis of their nutritive value. At the top of his list is cantaloupe, followed by watermelon, oranges, and honeydew melon.

Cantaloupe

Summer is the peak season, but good cantaloupes can usually be found in fall and spring at reasonable prices. The winter fruit is naturally more expensive, probably not as tasty, but still a good nutritional buy. Like most fruits, cantaloupes are picked green and shipped hard, but the ripening process is relatively swift. Appearance won't tell you much about ripeness. Press the stem end and sniff it, then press the whole melon; if there is a slight give, it is probably ripe. If not, store it at room temperature until it is and then put it in the refrigerator. Unused cut halves should be wrapped tightly, with the seeds left in, and kept in the refrigerator — the rule for all cut fruit.

Watermelon

This summer delight is one melon you can judge by looks, since most of us buy cut pieces. Obviously, the melon with the deep reddish color will taste a lot better and have more vitamin A than the paler early-season one.

Honeydews and Other Smooth-Skinned Melons

Somewhat less nutritious and considerably more expensive, honeydews, cranshaws, casabas, and the other more exotic melons are also considerably trickier to select. Honeydew especially is often hard as a rock, and this melon does take a long time to ripen — sometimes forever — from this state. Test for some give in the rind and hold the melon up to your ear and shake it; if you hear the seeds rattle, it's probably ripe.

Nectarines

These are a smooth-skinned, man-devised variety of peach, but not therefore to be less cherished. Nectarines have even more vitamin A and C than their parent fruit. Look for good, peachy color, and, as with most other fruits, store nectarines in the refrigerator once they've ripened.

Peaches

If you ever have the chance, buy this most delectable fruit from a roadside stand, in season and picked ripe. Even the New England varieties, with their fuzzy cheeks, are delicious under these circumstances — although they still can't be compared with a Georgia or Jersey peach fresh off the tree. Back in the real world of the supermarket, summer peaches are about as good as any fruit you can buy. Don't worry about their being hard as long as the background color is yellow; the green ones will shrivel rather than ripen. Ripen them in a brown paper bag at room temperature if you like, or in a pretty bowl so you won't forget they're around. When they are ripe, store them in the refrigerator. Peaches are a good source of vitamin A and some C.

Pears

One or more of the several varieties of pears are available year-round — Bartlett in the summer and Anjou, Bosc, and Comice in the winter. This is one fruit that doesn't do well in the refrigerator, so either buy pears when the flesh yields to the faintest touch or let them ripen at room temperature to that degree and eat them immediately. The core of the pear rots before the outer shell feels soft, so don't buy a lot of pears at one time.

Pineapple

This handsome, delicious, sweet but enigmatic fruit is difficult to select. Puerto Rico, Central and South America, and

Hawaii provide us with our supply. The ones flown in from Hawaii are the best tasting and most expensive; they tend to be ripe or overripe when you buy them. The ones grown south of the United States are usually shipped green, to ripen in the store. The time-honored way to test for ripeness is to give a little tug on one of the inner leaves; if it comes off in your hand, the pineapple is supposed to be ripe. Another test: smell the bottom; if there is no aroma, it isn't ripe. Even so, as any shopper knows, you can get stuck. If the pineapple is unripe, there's probably not much you can do, but if your "ripe" pineapple turns out to be rotten when you cut into it, take it back to the store. In general, look for the heaviest and largest pineapple in the bin, in shades of red and yellow rather than green.

A perfect pineapple is perfect eaten plain, but even a slightly unripe (and therefore slightly tasteless) one can be improved. Use it cut up with other fresh fruits, especially strawberries and melons, and pour a little orange liqueur or orange juice over everything.

If you buy canned pineapple, be sure to get the kind that is processed in its own juices.

Plums

Along with grapes, plums are a loser in the nutrient race, but only in comparison with other vitamin-rich fruit. Enjoy the various plums for their delicious taste and as a substitute for high-risk snacks and desserts.

Strawberries and Other Berries

Strawberries are a superb source of vitamin C. To add to their other delights, they are an exceedingly low-calorie dessert if you eat them in their pristine state. Select berries of moderate size; the overly large ones are usually tasteless. Although no store-bought berries can compare with the fresh-picked ones, you can do your part to ensure that you get your money's worth. Avoid a wet or stained container, and look at the bottom to be sure the berries aren't visibly weeping in their juices.

When you get home, separate the ripe ones (you may have to buy two cartons to get one full, ripe serving) and refrigerate them unwashed. Let the greenish white berries ripen at room temperature. If by the next day they're not ripe they should be thrown out or cooked for a few minutes with a little sugar and water to make a sauce.

Wash the ripe berries quickly just before you want to use them and *before* you take off the tops. If possible, remove the tops with a twist of your fingers rather than a knife.

All berries should be emptied from their cartons before they are stored in the refrigerator. With blueberries and raspberries, the problem is more likely to be overripe moldy berries than underripe ones. If you don't remove them, they'll infect the rest of the batch.

CHAPTER 13

Dry Staples:
Flour, Grains, Cereals,
and Legumes

Flour

The basic cereal grain of the West is wheat, and the flour from it — when unrefined — is an excellent source of complex carbohydrates, protein, vitamin E, the B vitamins, minerals, and fiber.

True, the protein is not complete, but the simple addition of a dairy product remedies this. Small wonder that wheat has been part of Western man's staple food for countless generations.

However, most of these important nutrients are found in the part of the grain kernel that today is usually discarded. As is true of all grains, wheat is composed of three parts. The germ is the most valuable source of nutrition; the outer layer, or bran, contains the roughage our body needs; the interior, or endosperm, is the one that yields only that smooth, white, starchy substance that is refined white flour.

This flour is so lacking in nutrients that the United States government, with its wartime powers in 1943, mandated that some of the nutrients be returned to flour, to try to safeguard the nation's health. This process, euphemistically known as enrichment, is now no longer compulsory, but many manufacturers do employ it. Far from being enriched, the flour and the goods made from it contain neither all the nutrients removed nor the fiber discarded from the outer layers. A rule of thumb is to choose an unrefined product preferably, then an enriched, and, lastly, unenriched flour products.

Following are the forms in which flours can be bought, and their uses.

Whole Wheat Flour

This is made from the entire grain — germ, bran, and all. It can be bought now in all supermarkets under the label of several of the largest companies. Since whole wheat flour is somewhat more attractive to cereal mites than white flour, store it in a large jar with a screw top or in the refrigerator.

Whole wheat flour can be substituted *in part* for white flour in all recipes except the most delicate cakes, adding two tablespoons less whole wheat per cup. We don't recommend using *all* whole wheat in either bread or cakes unless a very solid, heavy product is wanted.

White Flours

Unbleached flour. This is refined flour that has been spared the final step, a bleaching with chlorine. Unbleached flour is usually enriched and is the preferred choice for a white flour. Store as for whole wheat. Heckers and King Arthur are two good brands.

Enriched bleached flour. This is the most commonly used flour and is the next best choice in white flours.

Unenriched bleached flour. Seldom seen by the consumer, this is the flour most often used by bakeries.

Cake flour, self-rising, and plain. These are bleached and super-refined and are less common now that cake mixes have taken over the home baking market. You'll need to use cake flour for a delicate cake like an angel food, but unbleached white flour is fine for chocolate and other sturdy cakes.

Grains

Barley

This is a fine-tasting, nutritious grain *if* you get the correct variety. Whole grain barley is rich in protein, minerals, and fiber, but the pearled barley usually found in the super-market contains only a quarter of the protein and even less of the fiber and other nutrients than the unpolished. If you can't find whole grain barley or don't care to undertake the longer cooking that is necessary, look for Scotch rather than pearled barley. Fewer nutrients have been removed in Scotch barley, which makes it a good compromise.

Barley has more uses than the mushroom and beef soup it's generally known for. It's excellent in a turkey bone soup or in any vegetable combination soup where a thickening is needed. Time it according to which barley you're using so you don't overcook the vegetables while the grain is still not soft enough to eat.

Substitute barley for rice in a pilaf or risotto kind of dish — cook a cup of Scotch or pearled barley in two cups of chicken broth, add some grated onion, parsley, and season-ings. Either bake it or cook it on top of the stove.

Store barley on the shelf, in glass jars preferably.

Corn Meal

It used to be that white corn meal was found only in the South, yellow in the North. Now both can be bought in large supermarkets. There is little difference in food value, with the edge going to the yellow meal, particularly in vitamin A.

At best, corn meal is not a highly nutritious food. The only nutrients that are listed on the box of Quaker enriched and degerminated yellow corn meal are the four that have been added in the enrichment process — and the RDA percent-ages are quite insignificant.

In corn meal, unlike most grains, the enriched product is the better buy nutritionally, though water-ground meal makes a superior baking product. If you use corn meal for breading or any nonbaking use, buy the degerminated.

Water-ground corn meal should be kept in the refrigerator.

Corn bread or muffin mixes are probably the worst mixes on the market, oversweetened and highly chemical in taste.

Cracked Wheat

This is also known as bulgur or bulghour and is best found in a natural food store. In the supermarket, a packaged variety is sold as a pilaf, generally with added seasonings, and is always more expensive.

There are three sizes of cracked wheat, each with a different use:

The largest cut, sometimes called #3, is prepared by steaming, similarly to rice, and is the basis for a pilaf.

The middle size, #2, is used as a cooked cereal, similar to Wheatena-type brands.

Size #1 is a superb addition to bread, giving it that nutty, cracked wheat bite.

Wheat Germ

This is among the most convenient, most nutritious, most widely useful products in your larder. Keep a large jar on hand, but store it in the refrigerator. Wheat germ is an excellent source of thiamin and other B vitamins, vitamin E, and several minerals that are marginal in our diets — iron, zinc, magnesium, and copper. One-quarter cup provides the following percentages of the U.S. RDA for these minerals:

Iron	10 percent
Copper	15 percent
Magnesium	20 percent
Zinc	30 percent

Wheat germ is a "standard" food, so one brand starts out as good as another. However, since you want the freshest possible product, your supermarket's most popular brand is the best choice. Toasted wheat germ has a nice nutty taste, much better than the raw germ, which means you'll use it more liberally. Don't buy wheat germ with honey or sugar added.

Wheat germ is an easy habit to acquire. Add one-quarter cup to any hot or cold cereal. Use it to extend hamburgers or add it to meat loaf. Sprinkle it on cottage cheese, yogurt, or even ice cream.

Rye Flour

This is a good addition to some breads if used with a larger amount of white and whole wheat flours (they have the gluten rye lacks). Rye flour alone produces a sodden loaf and sticky hands. Rye flour is occasionally found in supermarkets, but more commonly in specialty or health food stores. It should be stored in the refrigerator.

Rice

PER 100 G	BROWN RICE	CONVERTED (ENRICHED)	WHITE (ENRICHED)	WHITE
Protein	7.5 g	7.4 g	6.7 g	6.7 g
Calcium	32 mg	60 mg	24 mg	24 mg
Phosphorus	221	200	94	94
Iron	1.6	2.9	2.9	0.8
Potassium	214	150	92	92
Sodium	9	9	5	5
Thiamin	0.34	0.44	0.44	0.07
Riboflavin	0.05	0.03	0.03	0.03
Niacin	4.7	3.5	3.5	1.6

Although brown rice is the most natural, and therefore the most nutritionally perfect form of rice, there is a good alternative for people who like their rice white: parboiled, or converted rice. Unlike regular white rice, which loses most of its germ and bran layer in processing, these elements are pretty well retained in the conversion method of processing rice.

Because converted rice is further "enriched," it has more of some nutrients, including iron, than brown rice — but it still has less of others. On a nutritional scale, brown rice rates first, followed in order by enriched converted rice, enriched white rice, and, at the bottom, instant rice.

Store white rice on a pantry shelf, brown rice in the refrigerator.

Soy Flour and Grits

Like the highly nutritious soybean from which they are ground, soy flour and grits (a larger particle than the flour) are high in complete protein and contain thiamin, riboflavin, niacin, and minerals. For people whose intake of animal products is low, for economic or humane reasons, these are excellent to combine with other flours in baking. All but the most dedicated vegetarian would probably want to blend flours to offset soy's strong flavor.

Soy flour and grits are to be found in health food stores, and they should be kept in the refrigerator.

Hot Cereals

Unrefined whole grain cereals are the first choice in nutrition, but even among hot cereals there are differences.

Wheat Cereals

Whole wheat cereal, under the brand name Wheatena and others, has the nutrients of the wheat grain, a nutty flavor, and best of all is as easy and almost as quick to make as any instant cereal.

If you strip away the bran layers and remove the germ from the wheat kernel, what remains is farina, the white, starchy endosperm. Farina cereals, therefore, have no bran and no wheat germ (the most concentrated source of nutrients in wheat) and are not nearly as nutritious as whole wheat, though they are usually enriched. They are also somewhat difficult to cook, with a decided tendency to lump; they aren't as good a choice as whole wheat cereals.

Oatmeal

Nutritionally, the order of preference is first, regular; second, quick-cooking; and third, instant. Irish steel-cut oats are high in nutrients, but they are fearfully expensive and, as a consequence, usually stale. They also require up to an hour of cooking.

Of all the hot cereals, regular oatmeal contains the most protein and thiamin, as well as fiber. It is also far easier to prepare than even the instructions on the Quaker box tell you. Mix the oatmeal and cold water (a little less than the amount called for) in a pot, according to how many you're serving, and go on with your other breakfast preparations, pausing only to stir the oatmeal and water for a few seconds (your bare hand is best) until the mixture is cloudy. Then, after five minutes or more of the oatmeal's simply sitting there, put a medium heat under it, let it simmer for three to five minutes, and you have the most delicious and creamy cereal you've ever eaten. Salt it if you wish; we don't.

About other oatmeals: quick-cooking isn't really any quicker, and far less tasty. Instant is another story. In addition to being steam-treated, rolled, cooked, and dried — all of which are death to heat-sensitive and water-soluble vitamins and minerals — it frequently has added salt. And tastes like library paste.

Cold Cereals

Significantly, when the cereal manufacturers advertise the nutritional goodness of their products, they scarcely mention the *cereal*, only the vitamins that have been added to it and the fact that it is eaten with milk. Nor do they mention that the chief additive is sugar.

No processed ready-to-eat cereal can compare nutritionally with a cooked whole grain cereal, but even in the real world, where cold cereal is a way of life, it is possible to be selective, to pick the best and avoid the worst. Here is what the manufacturers don't advertise:

The two most significant things to look for in a cold cereal are the amount of added sugar and the amount of processing the cereal has undergone. In both cases less is better, but be sure to consider both factors. Puffed cereals, with the least sugar, are the most highly processed. Some "natural" cereals, although lightly processed, are heavily sugared.

In the order of refinement, from least to most, shredded cereals are more lightly processed than flaked, and flaked are better than puffed, which are "shot from a gun" at temperatures high enough to remove most of their nutrients — puffed cereals are basically starch and air. If you match up this information with the sugar ratings in the table on the following pages, you can come up with enough variety in cereals to suit any taste.

For, of course, no one needs the variety of cereals on the market except manufacturers trying to beat out the competition for supermarket shelf space. In the end, it is the consumer who overpays, since many "different" cereals are nothing but expensive variations on an earlier model. Sugar Frosted Flakes are Corn Flakes with added sugar; you'll pay twice as much and eat more sugar than you would ordinarily have added to the Corn Flakes. Added coloring and sweeteners turn Kix (4.8 percent sugar) into Trix (35.9 percent sugar).

Total is Wheaties plus about 2 cents worth of vitamins, except that it costs the consumer 30 cents more — "a total ripoff," according to Michael Jacobson, executive director of the Center for Science in the Public Interest, which has formally complained about this cereal to the Federal Trade Commission.

Are "natural" cereals the answer? To the extent that they are made from whole grains, with seeds and nuts, they do have the natural vitamins and minerals and fiber that have been removed from most cereals and only partially replaced. Just don't equate natural with unsugared — as Jacobson points out, one-fifth of Quaker 100% Natural cereal is sugar; it should really be called 80% Natural. Granola is not only heavy on sugar (honey *is* sugar); the commercial varieties are more than 50 percent fat, including saturated fat.

One excellent, inexpensive, and tasty way to upgrade the quality of any cold cereal that your children eat is to add one-quarter cup of toasted wheat germ to every bowl of the processed product. There's only one ingredient on the label of a jar of wheat germ — wheat germ — but the list of natural vitamins and minerals is impressive.

In the mid-1970s, about six hundred health professionals, including doctors, dentists, and nutritionists, and more than twenty citizens' groups and professional organizations petitioned the Food and Drug Administration to force manufacturers to label cereal products containing more than 10 percent sugar with the actual percentage of sugar and the words "Frequent use contributes to tooth decay and other health problems." The petition was denied, but had it passed, only 17 of the 62 cereals in the following table, tested by the Department of Agriculture in 1979, would have been permitted to be sold without the warning. The letters following the name of the product refer to the manufacturers: General Foods (GF), General Mills (GM), Kellogg (K), Nabisco (N), Quaker Oats (QO), and Ralston-Purina (R-P).

PRODUCT	PERCENT SUGAR
Sugar Smacks (K)	56
Apple Jacks (K)	54.6
Froot Loops (K)	48
Raisin Bran (GF)	48
Sugar Corn Pops (K)	46
Super Sugar Crisp (GF)	46
Crazy Cow, chocolate (GM)	45.6
Corny Snaps (K)	45.5
Frosted Rice Krinkles (GF)	44
Frankenberry (GM)	43.7
Cookie Crisp, vanilla (R-P)	43.5
Cap'n Crunch, crunch berries (QO)	43.3
Cocoa Krispies (K)	43
Cocoa Pebbles (GF)	42.6
Fruity Pebbles (GF)	42.5
Lucky Charms (GM)	42.2

PRODUCT	PERCENT SUGAR
Cookie Crisp, chocolate (R-P)	41
Sugar Frosted Flakes of Corn (K)	41
Quisp (QO)	40.7
Crazy Cow, strawberry (GM)	40.1
Cookie Crisp, oatmeal (R-P)	40.1
Cap'n Crunch (QO)	40
Count Chocula (GM)	39.5
Alpha Bits (GF)	38
Honey Comb (GF)	37.2
Frosted Rice (K)	37
Trix (GM)	35.9
Cocoa Puffs (GM)	33.3
Cap'n Crunch, peanut butter (QO)	32.2
Golden Grahams (GM)	30
Cracklin' Bran (K)	29
Raisin Bran (K)	29
C. W. Post, raisin (GF)	29
C. W. Post (GF)	28.7
Frosted Mini Wheats (K)	26
Country Crisp (GF)	22
Life, cinnamon (QO)	21
100% Bran (N)	21
All Bran (K)	19
Fortified Oat Flakes (GF)	18.5
Life (QO)	16
Team (N)	14.1
40% Bran (GF)	13
Grape Nuts Flakes (GF)	13.3
Buckwheat (GM)	12.2
Product 19 (K)	9.9
Concentrate (K)	9.3
Total (GM)	8.3
Wheaties (GM)	8.2
Rice Krispies (K)	7.8
Grape Nuts (GF)	7
Special K (K)	5.4
Corn Flakes (K)	5.3
Post Toasties (GF)	5
Kix (GM)	4.8
Rice Chex (R-P)	4.4
Corn Chex (R-P)	4

PRODUCT	PERCENT SUGAR
Wheat Chex (R-P)	3.5
Cheerios (GM)	3
Shredded Wheat (N)	0.6
Puffed Wheat (QO)	0.5
Puffed Rice (QO)	0.1

One suggestion: you might want to copy the names and sugar percentages of the favorite brands in your house and post them on the refrigerator to let the children know what they are eating — consider it counter-advertising to combat what the manufacturers din in by way of television.

Dried Legumes

Legumes is a classier word than beans, but whatever you call them, any podded vegetables come under this category. Sometimes they are called peas. All of these dried legumes are excellent sources of protein, especially when eaten in combination with grains or dairy foods. The soybean is the only vegetable protein that is complete in itself.

There are about twenty-five different kinds of dried legumes, from the elegant imported flageolet, that delicate greenish white accompaniment to lamb in French cuisine, to the black-eyed peas of the American South and the garbanzo/ceci/chick peas of Italy, Spain, and Central America. There are yellow and green peas, split and whole peas, pigeon peas, lentils, and on and on.

Since most beans have some ethnic association, the best place to buy for variety and freshness is in ethnic markets. Lentils and dried lima beans are old standbys in Jewish cooking; along with split peas, they are the easiest beans to digest and a good place to start if you aren't used to eating beans. Small white beans with various names come from Scandinavian cooking. Look for pigeon peas and pinto beans in Hispanic neighborhoods. Some of these, along with pea beans, kidney beans, and others are also available in supermarkets. Soybeans are mostly found in health food stores.

Store dried beans, preferably in airtight jars, on the pantry shelf, except for soybeans, which belong in the refrig-

erator because of their fat content. Before using any legumes, wash them well in a bowl of water. Let the bits and
pieces of debris and the occasional discolored bean rise to
the top and discard them.

CHAPTER 14

Meats, Poultry, Fish

MAN HAS BEEN STRIVING to get and consume the flesh of one or more of the various other life forms for many, many eons. Meat in large amounts brings to mind not only gustatory pleasure but great bursts of energy, even feelings of well-being and prosperity. Restaurant menus flaunt individual servings of twenty-four-ounce steaks, three-pound lobsters, and a particularly American combo known winningly as surf 'n' turf, which comes spread across an eighteen-inch platter.

Our mythic tradition of good eating goes back to Henry VIII sitting before a haunch of beef — remember his gouty leg? — and twenty other courses. This need not be our standard today. There are ways of preparing food that will conform with health considerations, economic restraints, and even, possibly, social concerns. You don't have to be a zealot to feel good knowing you might have helped others to maintain life when you've merely abstained from overeating.

An excessive intake of animal, especially meat, products has two main dangers, both of which have been discussed earlier. First, the average American eats daily twice as much protein as the Food and Nutrition Board of the National Academy of Sciences recommends, and second, meat contains fat, particularly saturated fat, in amounts dangerous to our health. The Dietary Goals urge us to choose those meats, poultry, and fish that will reduce saturated fat intake and at the same time increase our complex carbohydrate foods. In

practice, this means cut down on fatty meat, partially substitute chicken and fish, and reduce the portion size of the
meat you do eat.

Beef

Beef is by far America's best seller. If rib roasts and steaks,
those nutritional and economic extravagances, are what
you're after, don't buy prime, the highest grade of beef. Yes,
it will have more marbling and be tenderer, but it will add
up to more fat in your system, even if you trim it well.
Choice and good grades are about equal in flavor, and you
can chew a little harder.

Round

This cut of beef is from the top of the leg, and while it has
a hefty surrounding layer of fat, it's not as marbled as rib
roast. Hence it's used mostly for braising (browned on top of
the stove with some liquid added and then covered). This
allows for the removal of the fat that has been rendered out
in cooking, particularly if the whole dish is prepared a day
prior to serving.

If you must have an oven roast, the eye of the round,
marinated in a wine or vinegar and oil mix and sliced thin
when served, is good. And for that occasion when nothing
but a steak will do, buy a plump flank steak, marinate as
above, broil, and serve sliced on a diagonal. Both of these
have far less fat than the more extravagant loin — porterhouse, filet, and T-bone — and sirloin cuts.

Chuck

A most useful cut of meat is the chuck, or shoulder. It
usually appears packaged as pot roast or sliced "steak." Buy
it in whichever form is cheaper in your store on a given day.
Sometimes a special on first cut chuck steaks will be 50
cents cheaper per pound than chuck pot roast from just

about the same part of the carcass. Compare the amount of fat, gristle, and bone for the money and choose accordingly. Do not buy boneless meat already cubed, labeled "stew meat." You're then paying for bones you don't have and fat you don't need in a cube size that's usually wrong for the meal. It takes about five minutes to cut the meat from the bone from either that labeled pot roast or steak, discard the fat (excellent for the birds), and slice the remaining meat exactly to your taste. That way you won't cut across a vein of fat but between it, thus eliminating the fatty deposits. Save the bones in the freezer for that day they will season a steaming pot of bean soup. It doesn't matter if a little meat clings to them; in fact it's all to the good.

Chopped Beef

Some states require the listing of fat percentage that can legally be incorporated in ground meat; other states permit the package to be referred to as being processed from a certain cut. In a simpler world, or perhaps still in custom butcher shops, actual pieces of identifiable meat were fed into the grinder before the eyes of the buyer. Faced with a supermarket package labeled ground sirloin, round, chuck, or simply ground meat, it is hard not to impute a certain amount of rascality to the loftier descriptions. One has visions of assorted scraps from who knows where chopped in with the token Designated Cut. Perhaps so. Retailers have not been above utilizing chemicals to simulate freshness by red coloring or to mask odors. It is to be hoped that these misdeeds are part of the past, but the mystery of what goes into the chopped meat remains. What it comes down to is this: Buy from a seemingly reputable store, and trust your eyes. The paler the package of chopped meat, the more fat, and this you want to avoid, particularly if you want to make hamburger patties. If, however, the dish you are preparing allows you to brown the meat first and discard the rendered fat, then, given equally fresh meat, decide according to the price.

Of course, if you own a classy kitchen appliance that will easily grind raw meat, then you'll really know what you're eating.

Veal and Lamb

Both of these have pretty much priced themselves off most American tables. Veal, the flesh of very young calves, has a lower fat content than other meats, but almost always requires additional fat in cooking. The exception is a top quality rump or leg roast.

Pork

Fresh pork roasts (loin, fresh ham) are fat-laden, but if you do want to have pork occasionally, buy chops or a whole piece — either loin or shoulder, whichever seems more reasonable at the time — and, after trimming off *all* the visible fat, cut it up small for use in a mixed dish, where a little bit of meat gives a lot of flavor.

Smoked or Cured Pork and Beef

Ham, bacon, hot dogs, sausages, bologna, salami, and so on. You've heard the bad news. The chemical chain is as follows: nitrate, which is harmless, converts to nitrite, which, interacting with the amines (found in beer, wine, cereals, tea, fish, and more than one thousand drugs) in the digestive process or in the presence of high heat, produces nitrosamines. The latter are clearly carcinogenic. Which is not to say that a serving of bacon or ham with grits and a cup of tea is inevitably going to cause cancer. What it does mean is that needless, dangerous substances are being added to your system. And who needs these uniformly high-fat foods anyway?

The chemicals used to cure, preserve, and make these products more appetizing looking are defended by the manufacturers for their role in preventing botulism toxins. What they don't add is that if more stringent sanitary procedures were followed, and if an almost indefinite shelf life were not demanded, there would be no such dangers. (See Chapter 10 on additives.)

Chicken

Chicken is the bright star in a sometimes dim firmament: lower in fat and cholesterol than red meat, versatile, and inexpensive. Stay with broilers and fryers (chickens under three pounds) and those with little visible fat. A preferred buying method is to select whole chickens and cut them to one's own needs, since there is then less handling and less flavor loss. This is particularly true if you intend to freeze the chicken after purchasing. However, if this seems a chore, or you're pressed for time, select an already cut one. Make sure the "cooled" chicken you buy isn't in fact frozen, since you then haven't the option to refreeze it.

The giblet package that comes with the chicken should not be discarded. Separate the liver from the other giblets and freeze the latter until you have a collection to make a good broth. Bits of the high-cholesterol livers can be used to garnish a grain dish.

Turkey

Fresh turkeys are making something of a comeback in some city markets. The choice of frozen or fresh is pretty much a pragmatic one. With nutritive values about equal, look for the size needed, price differential, and whether or not storage space is available in your freezer or refrigerator. After many years of experiments, we feel that flavor and moistness really depend on the correct roasting as much as on the choice of fresh or frozen. Of course, as for all frozen foods, check to make sure there are no signs of previous thawing and defrosting — the accumulated refrozen liquid can be felt under the plastic wrap.

A word of caution: Do not buy frozen turkeys injected ("basted," [*sic*]) with anything. These so-called butterballs are pumped with oil, usually saturated, sometimes with chemicals or sugar added. The flavors are suspect and the prices automatically higher. Do your own real basting. Your turkey shouldn't need a fix.

Turkey and Chicken Rolls

Avoid these dubious articles, usually found in the frozen food bins. Their food value is less than that of a comparable part of the poultry, and far more expensive. What convenience is offered is a poor trade-off for the inferior taste and nutrition.

Very Important Procedure: When handling all raw meats, but particularly chicken or turkey, be aware of the danger of salmonella, a baccillus that appears to be increasing in this country, and which grows easily in certain raw food. If you're unwrapping, cutting, or seasoning raw poultry, wash everything that has come in contact with it — the surface, knives, utensils, and your hands — with hot water and soap. There is no danger to the chicken or turkey itself, since the salmonella is killed in the cooking process. But some uncooked food, such as bread or salad, can pick up the bacilli on an unclean surface and cause a miserable sick stomach and head ailment. This should be kept in mind when shopping as well. Don't let the checker put any food in the same bag as raw poultry.

Fish

The various fresh ocean and inland water fish in our markets abound in things good for you — as long as they come from unpolluted waters. Fish is also about the most perishable of foods, not only subject to loss of nutrients but to contamination as well.

In buying fresh fish, avoid "prepared" items such as rolled and stuffed salmon, breaded shrimp, and deviled crabs. The less handling, the less chance of contamination. Fresh fish should be of good color, with no off odors, clear eyes (if bought whole), and firm flesh which should spring back after being pressed.

Concerning high levels of mercury in the very large fish high on the food chain, such as swordfish or tuna, there is little agreement on safe levels for human consumption of this mineral. Moderation would seem to be the sensible course; an occasional serving is probably harmless.

Frozen Fish

It ill behooves those of us fortunate to live within sight of the Atlantic Ocean to advise the purchase of only fresh fish. Of course frozen is a reasonable substitute when fresh can't be gotten, but be aware of the pitfalls.

Buy reputable brands, presented as simply as possible, that are firmly frozen with no evidence of prior defrosting (accumulated refrozen liquids in any part of the box) in a store where the temperature of the freezer is 0° to 5°F.

Avoid prepared, crumbed, breaded, or cooked fish in any form. They are more likely subject to contamination, and since their aim is to mask flavor they can begin with a less fresh product. The additives are legion.

Canned Fish

TUNA

In buying tuna fish there are a number of choices to be made according to quality, price, and amount of oil. In descending order of price and quality, these are: solid, chunk, flaked, and grated. Of the six species of tuna caught, only one, albacore, may be labeled as "white"; the other, "light meat," can actually be a deep brownish pink.

Additionally, tuna comes packed in either water or oil. Since the fat is extraneous to the fish, there is no reason to buy oil-packed tuna. If you do so, however, drain off the oil as thoroughly as possible; even so, some will adhere to the fish.

SALMON

Canned salmon is usually labeled according to color, from red to pale pink, and the name of the species. In descending price order these are red, sockeye; red, chinook or king; medium red, silver or coho; pink, chum or keta. There is only one packing style, a kind of natural broth in which the fish is processed. This can be used in a casserole or chowder, to receive all the nutrients you paid for. The deeper the red color, the higher the fat content.

SARDINES

These tiny fish are canned in this country and abroad, packed as skinned and boned or plain. If the tiny bones are eaten, they are a source of calcium and fluorine. Drain oil-packed sardines to avoid unnecessary fat.

CHAPTER 15

Dairy Products and Substitutes

BUTTERFAT, ONCE THE SYMBOL of the best in taste and nutrition in milk and milk products, from butter to cheese to heavy whipping cream, is a casualty of this cholesterol-conscious age. With the publication of *Dietary Goals for the United States* and its linking of saturated fats to certain cancers as well as heart disease, it becomes more important than ever to select dairy products wisely. This certainly doesn't imply that we eliminate these foods from our diet — they are our primary source of calcium and vitamin D, an excellent source of protein, and a good source of vitamins A and B$_2$ — but it does suggest that we may have to make some modifications in the kinds of dairy foods we eat, especially the ones we eat on a regular basis. Single-product solutions are not the answer, as the margarine manufacturers would have us believe. It does no good to put margarine on your bread if you top it with cream cheese.

Butter or Margarine

The original appeal of margarine was that it was cheaper than butter. It's still cheaper, but the magic word behind its success in recent years (it has overtaken butter in sales) is *polyunsaturated*. If concern over saturated fat and cholesterol is your reason for eating margarine, here are some guidelines to help you achieve your goals.

Butter is butter, but margarine is made up of a number of

things, including additives. In two respects, butter and margarine are the same — they have the same number of calories and the same amount of total fat. Exceptions are "imitation" diet margarines in which water replaces some of the fat for a saving of half the calories.

Where margarine differs significantly from butter is in the amount of saturated fat. Butter is more than half saturated fat; margarines are a combination of saturated and polyunsaturated fats, and the proportions vary widely among different brands.

Margarines are made from liquid vegetable oils, and different oils have different proportions of polyunsaturated to saturated fats. (Please read about oils and margarines in Chapter 2.) However, to make the margarine hard enough to remain solid at room temperature, some of the liquid oil must be hydrogenated — in effect, saturated. This suggests a compromise for the person who likes the taste of butter but wants the polyunsaturated fat in vegetable oil. Instead of using margarine for eating and cooking, use butter sparingly on your bread and polyunsaturated vegetable oil for cooking and baking.

The best (and most expensive) margarines are those with the highest ratio of polyunsaturated to saturated fats — generally, the ones that have "liquid" corn or safflower oil as the first ingredient and partially hydrogenated corn or safflower oil as the second. Fleischmann's, for instance, has 4 grams of polyunsaturated fat and 2 grams of saturated, a ratio of 2 to 1. This is the ratio to aim for. Margarines made of soy oil or cottonseed oil generally have a poor ratio of polyunsaturated to saturated fat.

When selecting margarines, read the nutritional information on the outside of the package. Buy the one that has at least twice as much polyunsaturated as saturated fat. Soft or tub margarines, which require less hydrogenation (since they don't have to hold their shape), as a rule have the best ratios of polyunsaturated to saturated fat.

Whipped margarines and imitation diet margarines have fewer calories and less total fat than regular stick or tub margarines. However, they are unsatisfactory for cooking;

when heated, they tend to get foamy or lumpy, or the oil and water in the imitation types separate.

Milk

Unlike butter, there are different kinds of "real" milk that offer a choice for people who want to cut down on saturated fat and cholesterol. Except for young children, the Dietary Goals suggest that our choice be a low-fat or nonfat milk. Since all milk has about the same amount of protein, as the percentage of fat is lowered, the protein percentage is raised. The other nutrients, including calcium, remain the same and nothing is lost but the fat and cholesterol. Be sure to buy "enriched" milk with vitamin D and, usually, A added. Vitamin C is also added to some milk, but this is not a necessary enrichment for anyone who drinks a glass of orange juice or its equivalent.

LIQUID MILK IN 8-OUNCE PORTIONS	CALORIES	TOTAL FAT (G)	SATURATED FAT (G)	CHOLESTEROL (MG)
Whole	157	8.9	5.0	35
2% fat	121	4.7	2.9	18
1% fat	102	2.6	1.6	10
Skim	86	0.44	0.28	4

From U.S. Department of Agriculture Handbook #8–1

Dry Milk

Dried whole milk reconstitutes to a liquid that corresponds nutritionally very well to whole skim milk. It is, appropriately, fortified with vitamins A and D. It is invaluable for both cooking and baking, and simply adding it to other foods boosts their nutrition value. If you add some nonfat dry milk to liquid skim milk, you'll get a richer tasting, higher protein product without the fat of whole milk. More economical too.

Dry skim milk is marketed by several "name" firms, but also under store brands, and these are identical and cheaper. Two packaging types are available, a pour-spout box and one in which measured portions are in envelopes, each making a quart of liquid. We think the pour-spout box offers more flexibility.

Cheese

Like other dairy products, cheese is an excellent source of protein and calcium and unfortunately — except for cottage cheese — saturated fat. It is also, again except for cottage cheese, a highly caloric food. In the following table, the values are given for 1-ounce portions. One ounce isn't very much. The next time you buy a pound of cheese, cut it into sixteen pieces to get an idea of what a 1-ounce piece looks like.

CHEESE (1 OUNCE)	CALORIES	PROTEIN (G)	TOTAL FAT (G)	SATURATED FAT (G)	CHOLESTEROL (MG)
Blue	100	6.0	8.1	5.3	21
Camembert	85	5.6	6.8	4.3	20
Cheddar	114	7.0	9.4	5.9	30
Fontina	110	7.2	8.8	5.4	33
Cream cheese	99	2.1	9.9	6.2	31

From U.S. Department of Agriculture Handbook #8–1

Cheese is one of our most concentrated sources of saturated fat. It is one thing to eat cheese as a part of a meal, instead of meat. The trouble for most of us is that we nibble on cheese as a snack food — in addition to all the other saturated fats we consume each day.

Hard cheeses are sold in two main forms, natural and processed, with processed far outselling the natural in the stores.

Simple "pasteurized process cheese" differs from natural cheese in that it has been treated with heat. It loses a lot in taste but not very much in nutrients. Further down the processing line, though, we get "processed cheese food" and "processed cheese spread." These products suffer substantial losses in protein, calcium, and other minerals and nutrients. They are a poor buy for your nutritional dollar.

As for "imitation cheeses" with "half the calories" of cheese, cardboard has even fewer, and it probably has fewer additives too.

Cottage Cheese

Cottage cheese is an entirely different story. It has all the virtues of cheese with few of the drawbacks. You can buy it creamed or low-fat, natural or with additives, small curd or large curd. There is a remarkable variation in taste among the different brands, so if you haven't yet found one you really like, shop around. This is a food to have on hand at all times; for lunches, to spread on toast instead of cream cheese, to snack on, and even to use in cooking. Try it in pancakes, stirred into hot noodles, or as a low-calorie substitute for ricotta in pasta dishes.

For breakfast, instead of cold cereal or eggs, serve cottage cheese with cut up fruit topped with wheat germ. As a luncheon salad it goes well with tomatoes, cucumbers, or any other raw vegetable.

COTTAGE CHEESE (4 OUNCES)	CALO-RIES	PROTEIN (G)	TOTAL FAT (G)	SATU-RATED FAT (G)	CHOLES-TEROL (MG)
Creamed cottage cheese (4% fat)	117	14.1	5.1	3.2	13
Cottage cheese (2% fat)	101	15.5	2.2	1.4	9
Cottage cheese (1% fat)	82	14.0	1.1	0.73	5
Ricotta (part skim milk)	171	14.1	9.8	6.1	38

From U.S. Department of Agriculture Handbook #8–1

Yogurt

Although there's considerable skepticism about the claim that the bacillus in yogurt is what's keeping all those Russian Georgians doing the sword dance at age 132, yogurt is as good a food, and no better, than the milk from which it derives.

You can buy yogurt made from whole or skim milk, with or without additives. The amount of fat and the number of calories will only reflect the kind of milk it was made from.

Flavored yogurt, or yogurt with added fruit preserves, is by no means a low-calorie food, since it may have as much as 100 calories more than the plain variety.

Plain yogurt is an excellent substitute, in eating and cooking, for sour cream, as the following table indicates.

YOGURT (8 OUNCES)	CALO- RIES	PROTEIN (G)	TOTAL FAT (G)	SATU- RATED FAT (G)	CHOLES- TEROL (MG)
Yogurt, whole milk, plain	139	8	7.38	4.76	29
Yogurt, low- fat, plain (with added solids)	144	12	3.52	2.27	14
Yogurt, skim milk, plain	127	13	0.41	0.26	4
Yogurt, low- fat, fruit	231	10	2.45	1.58	10
Sour cream	493	7	48.21	30.01	102

If you do want to use sour cream, thin it by a third with skim milk, let it blend for a few minutes, and then use it as you would whole sour cream. It will, of course, be more of a liquid and can't be "exchanged" in delicate cake baking. It is useful in cooking when you don't want to substitute yogurt.

Ice Cream and Ice Milk

These vary in calories, fat, and sugar content almost as much as in flavors. If you're confused about the difference between some of the frozen desserts, these are the specifications:

Luxury brand ice creams are those with 16 percent butterfat and consequently usually require less sugar for taste appeal. An 8-ounce serving of French vanilla of this quality is 377 calories (soft serve) or 349 (hardened). Some of the custard ice creams also include eggs, so cholesterol is an added hazard.

Regular ice cream, with about 10 percent fat, has 269 calories to an 8-ounce serving of vanilla flavor. Some of the cheaper regular ice creams will contain somewhat less cream and more sugar, as well as being loaded with artificial flavors.

Ice milk contains between 2 and 7 percent milkfat, and the same 8 ounces of vanilla flavored ice milk contains 184 calories.

Sherbet is a frozen dessert that may contain fruit, usually fruit flavoring, and only 1 to 2 percent milkfat. Its main ingredient is sugar, and of all the frozen desserts sherbet comes closest to junk food. An 8-ounce cup is 270 calories.

All frozen desserts should be stored in your freezer and used within a few weeks, preferably. Before putting an open carton back in the freezer, cover the surface with a protective wrap to avoid unpleasant crystallization.

CHAPTER 16

Snack Foods

WHEN IT COMES TO dietary risks, the snack aisles of the supermarket are mined with booby traps. If it were possible to improve the dietary habits of a lifetime in one single step, that step would be to avoid buying crackers, cookies, candy, chips, pretzels, packaged pastries — and all the colas and other sodas needed to wash them down. Of all the foods we eat, these have simultaneously the least nutrients and the most sugar, salt, fat, and artificial additives.

Since snacking is a way of life — from the eleven o'clock coffee break, mid-afternoon pick-up, and the before bedtime nightcap, to almost constant TV munching, to the refrigerator raids of a fifteen-year-old home from school — it isn't enough to eliminate junk snacks. The trick is to replace them with real foods. And to take a lesson from the food manufacturers who know that the most easily eaten foods, the ones that take no more effort than dipping a hand into a package, are the ones that will be consumed in quantity.

In other words, load up your refrigerator with ready-to-eat snacks. If raw vegetables have to be prepared from scratch they'll be passed by, but if you always have a covered container in the front of the refrigerator filled with a variety of crisp vegetables — carrots, celery, sweet green and red peppers, zucchini, cherry tomatoes, young peas (shelled or in the pod), radishes, broccoli, string beans, even leaves of lettuce or spinach — they will be eaten. Especially if you also have handy in the refrigerator a jar of tangy dressing made of oil and vinegar, or yogurt, or puréed spiced cottage cheese.

At the same time that you make good snacks convenient to eat, try to make the others less so. Nuts, although they tend to be fatty, are nutritious if eaten without salt and in moderation. Instead of a bowl of salted, shelled nuts, keep a supply of nuts in the shell; the exercise of shelling will slow down the intake while keeping you busy (which is part of the reason we snack).

Toasted sunflower seeds are a highly nutritious substitute for nuts. Don't buy the expensive salty ones in the tiny packages sold in the supermarkets, though. You can buy them by the pound for far less money, without the salt, in a natural food store. While you are there, experiment with small amounts of pumpkin or other seeds.

Although store-bought cookies are a nutritional risk, you certainly don't have to deprive a child of a cookie and a glass of milk. You'll find recipes for nutritious, unadulterated cookies in Chapter 23. Make up a batch and keep them in the freezer in small packages. Better yet, let the children make them themselves — with the clear understanding that the whole recipe is not for one snack.

Most store-bought crackers are every bit as bad as packaged cookies, but there are a few that aren't full of salt, sugar, fats, and additives. Read the labels.

Consider the virtues of whole wheat bread, instead of crackers, as a snack food. For a child, especially, bread and peanut butter and a glass of milk is a snack that is high in protein, vitamins, and minerals.

Fresh homemade popcorn is an excellent snack food. Eaten warm, it doesn't even need salt or margarine, but if you use these additions, use a very light hand.

As a traditional snack food, hard cheese, unfortunately, has some serious drawbacks, as we saw in the last chapter. Cottage cheese has none and can be eaten at any time, alone, with fruit, or spread on a piece of whole wheat bread. Plain yogurt is another food to consider as a staple snack if you like the taste.

For a liquid accompaniment to snacking, milk and real

fruit juices are the best possible choices. Soft drinks are the worst.

When you buy ice cream, don't try to make a mini–ice cream parlor of your freezer. Unlimited quantities are an invitation to large and frequent helpings. Buy one flavor at a time of ice milk, not ice cream, and let it be considered an occasional treat.

Do just the opposite with the best of all snack foods, fresh fruit. Keep your refrigerator well stocked with fruit, and make sure that some pieces are out on the table where they can't be overlooked when hunger strikes. Buy every kind of fruit you can find, even if it seems expensive. Compared to what you get, and don't get, in packaged snack foods, even luxury fruit is a bargain. Use the money you save on junk food for fruit.

Dried fruit is a superior snack food because of its concentrated sweetness and nutrients. It does have two drawbacks: it is highly caloric and sticky, which means that the sugar remains between the teeth. Children, especially, who eat dried fruit should be encouraged to brush their teeth afterward.

It's a good idea to pair dried fruit with fresh; for instance, a few raisins with a crisp apple or an orange sliced with a cut up date or two.

A number of nutritionists have developed systems for scoring foods according to their plus and minus nutritional components, a kind of simplified shorthand. Different systems include different factors, but the overall score for a food usually gives a good picture of what you want to know. Following are two different, handy ratings for snack foods. Both are included to cover the widest selection of snacks. Where the same foods are included in both lists, it is interesting to note that even though different systems were used, the foods generally receive the same relative scores.

In *The Complete Food Handbook*, authors Rodger P. Doyle and James L. Redding assign plus points for vitamins, minerals, and fiber, and minus points for "questionable" additives such as artificial flavor and coloring, refined flour, and excessive salt. The arbitrary ratings run from a possible

+100 to −50. While we do not agree with Doyle and Redding's equating some unnecessary but harmless additives with truly dangerous amounts of sugar, salt, and fat, it is a generally useful assessment.

Orange	80	Triscuits	10
Banana	70	Pringles potato chips	0
Peanuts	50	Doritos tortilla chips	0
Plain yogurt	40	Orange sherbet	−10
Ry Krisp	40	Fritos corn chips	−10
Ice cream 10% fat	40	Hostess Twinkies	−10
Hunt's Snack Pack Fruit Cup	40	Homemade chocolate chip cookies	−10
Apple with skin	40	Hunt's Snack Pack chocolate pudding	−10
Pizza with sausage	40		
Cheddar cheese	30	Graham crackers	−20
Swiss-style strawberry yogurt	20	Salted soda crackers	−20
Raisins	10	Doughnut	−30
Milk chocolate	10	Cola	−50
Potato chips	10	Popsicle	−50

In the scoring system worked out in *Nutritional Scoreboard* by Dr. Michael Jacobson of the Center for Science in the Public Interest, the formula is arrived at by assigning plus numbers to protein, naturally occurring carbohydrates (including starch, fiber, and natural sugars), certain vitamins and minerals, and unsaturated fat. Minus numbers are given to added sugar and corn syrup, saturated fat, and a high overall fat content. There is no arbitrary upper or lower limit.

Granola and milk	45	Cashews	24
Sunflower seeds	44	Walnuts	17
Almonds	31	Raisins	13
Peach	29	Apple	12
Peanuts	25	Triscuits	9
Granola	25	Potato chips	8

Popcorn (no butter)	6	Milky Way candy bar	−33
Oatmeal cookie	−4	M&M's candy	−33
Sandwich cookie	−7	Cracker Jacks	−39
Snickers candy bar	−23	Hostess Sno-Ball	−44
Mars almond candy		Popsicle	−45
bar	−27	3 Musketeers candy	
Milk chocolate	−27	bar	−55
Brownie	−30	Chuckles candy	−74

Part III

Recipes and Cooking Procedures

CHAPTER 17

Homemade Convenience Foods

CONVENIENCE. We all seek it, but Americans have been beguiled into accepting almost any product that promises to save time and/or work. For the dubious claims of "convenience foods" we've spent large sums of money, but in so doing have accepted many products injurious to our health.

In this chapter we'd like to suggest a middle-of-the-road approach. Five concerns are present in the cooking process: nutrition, taste, time, work, and money. By going along with some, but not all, of the highly processed foods you can indeed save some time and work, though few would quarrel that at the same time you lose nutrition, taste, and money. There *are* ways to achieve a balance of all five without returning to great-grandma's kitchen routines; a little ingenuity goes a long way.

We include here some easy substitutes for a few of the convenience products and some techniques that will add savor to your meals, painlessly and nutritionally.

• *Basic Muffin and Pancake Mix* •

- 8 cups unbleached white flour (part whole wheat can be used)
- 3 tablespoons plus 1 teaspoon baking powder
- 2 teaspoons salt
- 1 cup sugar
- 1⅓ cups dry skim milk

½   cup wheat germ
2   teaspoons cinnamon

In a large bowl stir all the ingredients lightly but thoroughly. Store the mix in a covered container. Stir it gently each time some of the mix is removed.

• *Baked Muffins* •
Makes 12 large or 16 medium muffins

These foolproof muffins are sweet enough for a simple dessert, especially if they're served warm.

2¾   cups Basic Muffin and Pancake Mix
1   cup water
1   egg, beaten
⅓   cup sunflower or corn oil
Optional additions:
½   cup raisins
½   cup dates, cut up
¾   cup grated or thinly sliced apples, plus ½ teaspoon cinnamon
½   cup berries, drained if frozen
1   teaspoon grated orange peel (good with any addition)

1. Stir the muffin mix in the large container and remove 2¾ cups to a large bowl. Do not pack down when measuring the mix.
2. Combine the water, egg, and oil, and stir the liquids into the dry mix just enough to dampen all the dry ingredients. The batter should not be completely smooth.
3. Stir in any of the optional additions, fill well-greased muffin tins ⅔ full, and bake in preheated oven at 400° for about 20–25 minutes.

• *Pancakes* •
Serves 4

1½   cups Basic Muffin and Pancake Mix
1   egg, well beaten

3   tablespoons melted margarine or corn oil
⅔   cup liquid low-fat or skim milk
½   cup water

1. Stir the mix in the container and remove 1½ cups to a large bowl.

2. Add the remaining ingredients, pour them into the dry mix, and combine with a few strokes. If the batter seems too thick, add a little more milk, but do not beat out all the lumps. If desired, the batter can be prepared several hours in advance and refrigerated.

3. Heat a griddle and grease it lightly. It is hot enough when a drop of water sizzles. Drop the batter by spoonfuls onto the griddle. Turn each pancake when the top side is bubbly. Serve as soon as the second side is brown.

Variation: For a dessert pancake, thin the batter with a tablespoon or so of milk, add 1 teaspoon each of grated orange and lemon rind, and ½ cup of thinly sliced (or grated) sweet apples (McIntosh are good) or drained blueberries.

• *Cornell Nutrition Booster, Adapted* •

Some thirty years ago nutritionists at Cornell University produced a formula that raised significantly the protein level of baked goods — breads particularly. The original formula called for soy flour and brewer's yeast, which have a strong taste. Many people found the flavor unpleasant and rejected the formula entirely. We suggest you try it both with and without the soy flour and yeast.

Note: These ingredients are to be added to traditional recipes. Those given in this book have already been adapted.

2   tablespoons dry milk
1½ tablespoons wheat germ
1   tablespoon soy flour
1   teaspoon brewer's yeast

Stir the ingredients together and place in the bottom of the cup before measuring flour for bread, muffins, or even some cookie recipes.

Plain and Flavored Bread Crumbs

Keep a jar or bag of bread ends in the refrigerator or freezer. Whir the pieces in a blender before using, or keep them on hand by preparing a jarful in advance. Store in the refrigerator. If soft crumbs are wanted for a particular dish, whir up 2 slices of fresh bread for a cupful.

Don't make cheese-flavored crumbs ahead of time because the flavor and freshness of the cheese will flag. Add cheese to crumbs only as needed.

The purpose of Shake 'n Bake–type crumb breadings is to mask the taste of chicken with a heavily sweetened, chemicaled, and needlessly expensive mixture. They are meant primarily for "oven-fried" chicken or chops, a process that often uses more fat than does frying. Instead, follow the recipe for broiled chicken on page 179. Bake the chicken at 400° for almost an hour, basting occasionally.

For variety, if you want to use a crumb type breading without the extra sugar and fat in the commercial product, try this two-step process.

• *Crumbs for Three Chickens* •

3   cups bread crumbs, preferably your own, but otherwise the unseasoned packaged kind
¼   cup whole wheat flour
3   tablespoons wheat germ
¼   teaspoon marjoram, thyme, or sage
2   teaspoons pepper
1   teaspoon salt
1   teaspoon grated lemon or lime rind

Mix all the ingredients well, and store, covered, in the refrigerator.

• Baked, Crumbed Chicken •

1. To use the crumb mixture for one chicken, stir it well and take out one heaping cupful. Put it in a large flat dish and reserve.

2. Place the cut up chicken in a shallow baking dish.

3. Combine 3 tablespoons Garlic-Flavored Oil (see page 153) and 3 tablespoons Garlic-Flavored Wine Vinegar, and rub it into the chicken pieces. Let them stand about 20 minutes or more.

4. Dip the chicken pieces into the crumbs, patting them in with your hands.

5. Return the chicken pieces to the baking pan, spoon over any excess marinade, and bake at 400° for about an hour.

Salad Dressing

The list of reasons to substitute your own salad dressings for the bottled stuff is longer than the chemical ingredients in French Diet Lite, but avoiding sugar and additives is high on the list. Once your taste buds get desugared you'll wonder how you ever thought bottled dressings were palatable.

• French Dressing, Simon Pure •

The true French dressing is neither made ahead of time nor premixed; instead, the ingredients are added to the salad individually.

3 to 4   parts Garlic-Flavored Oil, or half olive oil
    1   part Garlic-Flavored Wine Vinegar
         pepper and salt to taste

Sprinkle the oil, then the vinegar, and finally the salt and fresh-ground pepper over well-drained greens. Turn gently and serve.

• *French Dressing, Adapted* •

½	teaspoon dry mustard
¼ to ⅓	cup Garlic-Flavored Wine Vinegar
1	cup Garlic-Flavored Oil
	pepper and salt
½	teaspoon sugar (optional, if you must)

Place the dry mustard in a pint-sized screw-top container, and stir in a little vinegar to make a paste. Then add the other ingredients. Store on the pantry shelf and shake well before using.

• *Italian Dressing, Adapted* •

1	cup Garlic-Flavored Oil
⅓	cup Garlic-Flavored Wine Vinegar
½	teaspoon dried oregano or dried sweet basil

Follow directions for French Dressing, Adapted. Store on the pantry shelf and shake well before using.

• *Creamy Salad Dressing* •

This dressing can be stored in a jar in the refrigerator for several days — up to a week if the cottage cheese is very fresh.

1	cup cottage cheese, low-fat or regular
¼	cup low-fat liquid milk
2	teaspoons onion, cut up
1	tablespoon lemon juice or Garlic-Flavored Wine Vinegar
	pepper and salt to taste
¼	cup mayonnaise or yogurt, optional

Combine the cottage cheese, milk, lemon juice, and onion in a blender and whir until it is smooth. If dressing is not liquid enough for your taste, add a little more milk. Season with pepper and salt. Fold in the yogurt or mayonnaise if desired.

Additional creamy salad dressings can be made from the Dips on page 163 by increasing the liquids.

• Garlic-Flavored Oil and Garlic-Flavored Wine Vinegar •

Both the oil and the vinegar can be used in salad dressings and in marinades. The oil can be used in sautéing vegetables for soup or a mixed dish. Both are *real* conveniences, no stronger than garlic powder, and with a more natural taste.

GARLIC-FLAVORED OIL

2   large cloves garlic
1   pint corn oil

Cut the garlic cloves in half and place them in a pint-sized screw-top container. Add the oil.

If the oil is kept longer than three or four weeks remove the garlic.

GARLIC-FLAVORED WINE VINEGAR

Follow the same procedure as with the oil, though you may not wish to make a full pint at one time.

Dessert

• Freezer or Refrigerator Cookie Roll •
Makes about 110 cookies, according to thickness

This is a delicious cookie without the excessive sugar, saturated fat, and additives of the store-bought product. It's a lot cheaper too.

¾   cup margarine
1½ cups sugar (1¼ cups if the cinnamon sugar topping is
       used; see Variations)

¼   cup nonfat dry milk
¼   cup sunflower or corn oil
1   egg plus 1 egg white
1   tablespoon grated orange peel or 1 teaspoon lemon
      peel
1   teaspoon vanilla extract
½   teaspoon salt
4   cups white unbleached flour

1. Cream the sugar, margarine, and dry milk in the large bowl of an electric mixer, if available, or by hand, and mix until fluffy. Add the oil, egg, and egg white, and beat for another minute.

2. Stir in the grated orange peel and vanilla.

3. Add the flour and salt with a minimum of beating. The last cupful or so should be worked in with a spoon or your hands.

4. Shape the batter into rolls about 1½ or 2 inches in diameter and 8 inches in length. Wrap individually in freezer paper and store in freezer until wanted.

Instead of freezing, one or more of the rolls can be stored in the refrigerator if used within three or four days.

To use the frozen rolls, remove from the freezer, unwrap, and slice the cookies about ¼ inch thick. Sprinkle on a topping if you wish.

Place the sliced cookies on a greased tin and bake in 400° pre-heated oven for about 12 minutes or until light brown. Watch carefully to prevent burning, especially if the cookies are sliced thinner than ¼ inch.

Variations: For one 8-inch bar mix 1½ tablespoons of sugar and ¾ teaspoon of cinnamon, or combine ¼ cup chopped nuts and 1 tablespoon wheat germ. Sprinkle on top of the sliced cookies before baking.

Note: Almost any cookie recipe can be adapted to refrigerator-freezer cookie rolls; simply cut down the liquid ingredients. The oatmeal cookie recipe on page 246 freezes particularly well in this manner, but the cookies may need to be cut a trifle thicker than ¼ inch.

• *Whipped Topping* •
Makes 2 cups

This can't be confused with heavy whipping cream, but it tastes no worse than Cool Whip and has the advantage of being made of real food ingredients. This cannot be made more than an hour or so in advance or it will separate.

½   cup, minus 2 tablespoons, *iced* (almost frozen is best) water
½   cup dry skim milk
1½ tablespoons sugar
1   teaspoon lemon juice

1. Place the water in a bowl in the refrigerator or freezer until it is very cold (almost frozen is best).
2. Add the skim milk and beat at high speed with an electric mixer or by hand for 2 or 3 minutes, until the mixture is stiff enough to hold a peak.
3. Fold in the sugar and lemon juice and beat for a few more seconds. Chill in the refrigerator for half an hour or longer, or in the freezer for about 10 minutes.

CHAPTER 18

Appetizers

NOT THAT MOST OF US need to stimulate our appetite — but "a little something before dinner" has become an institution, whether it's a carrot stick and cottage cheese while you're fixing the meal or something more elaborate.

When company comes, two or twenty, you certainly want to be hospitable, warm, gracious, and little showoffy. The big thing is to present an elegant rather than extravagant table, with food that enhances your guests' health, not their waistlines. Vegetable appetizers are an ideal choice, but they need not be limited to the ubiquitous raw vegetables with a dip that we're now calling crudités. Some of the recipes in this chapter can double for fancy lunch dishes as well.

• *Vegetables à la Grecque* •
Serves 4

1. Clean and prepare about 2½ cups of vegetables. Good choices are small onions, string beans, carrots, mushrooms, and celery, but others can be used. Slice the large vegetables, and leave the small ones, mushrooms especially, whole.

2. Simmer the following mixture for 10 minutes in a non-aluminum pan.

1¾   cups water
½   cup onion, roughly cut
½   cup celery, sliced

6   sprigs parsley, Italian preferably
1   large or 2 small cloves garlic, cut in half
1   bay leaf
1   teaspoon whole peppercorns
    pinch of thyme
    pepper and salt

3. Add and simmer for 2 minutes more:

⅓   cup wine vinegar
⅓   cup corn or sunflower oil

4. Strain off all the ingredients from the broth and discard them.

5. Add the vegetables according to their cooking time, being careful not to overcook. Use these times as your guide: small onions and string beans — 15 to 20 minutes; carrots and celery — 10 to 15 minutes, according to thickness; mushrooms — 6 to 8 minutes.

When all the vegetables are crisply done, taste one for seasoning and correct if necessary with additional pepper and salt. Chill the mixture in a covered bowl. If there is excess broth, set it aside and use it another time as a raw vegetable dressing; it can keep in the refrigerator for weeks. Serve well chilled or at room temperature, with additional cut up parsley.

• *Grilled Green or Red Sweet Pepper* •

1. Remove the skin from as many peppers as you wish. You can do this by putting a fork in the pepper and rotating it over a gas flame, as if you were toasting marshmallows. If you have an electric stove or are skinning a number of peppers, put them on a foil-covered flat pan close to the heating element of the broiler. Turn the peppers to achieve a fairly even burn.

2. Run the peppers quickly under a light stream of water to remove the burnt skin. They will look splotchy. Discard the seeds and stem.

3. Cut the peppers lengthwise into strips, and marinate

them for at least an hour in a dressing of two parts Garlic-Flavored Oil and one part Garlic-Flavored Wine Vinegar. These are best eaten the same day, though they will keep longer.

A short cut: Use bottled pimientos, but *not* the thick-skinned kind, instead of grilling the peppers.

• *Radishes au Printemps* •

When radishes are in season, in late spring and summer, they are often sold with their green tops fresh and intact. Serve them French-style in a white bowl: with a few ice cubes underneath, the green tops forming a little bouquet, and the red showing through. The classic accompaniments to this are a dish of sweet butter and a saltcellar. Our compromise is Herbed Cottage Cheese, on page 162, omitting radishes from the mixture.

• *Stuffed Mushrooms* •
Serves 4

This hot appetizer is adapted from a very buttery original.

8 or 10	large mushrooms
3	tablespoons Garlic-Flavored Oil
1	cup bread crumbs
¼	cup wheat germ
2	tablespoons grated Parmesan cheese
3	tablespoons minced or grated onion
3	tablespoons minced parsley, Italian preferably
	pepper and salt

1. Remove the stems (save them for other dishes) and clean the mushrooms, using little or no water if possible.

2. Brush the mushrooms with two-thirds of the oil.

3. Combine all the other ingredients except the reserved oil and stuff the mushrooms lightly.

4. Drizzle the remaining oil over the tops, place the mushrooms on a foil-covered baking sheet, and either broil

for about 10 minutes or bake at 375° for about 15 minutes until lightly browned. Serve immediately or the mushrooms will shrivel.

• *Ratatouille* •
Serves 6 to 8, as an appetizer

¼	cup oil
1	large eggplant, about 1½ pounds
2 to 4	zucchini, medium size
2	cups canned tomatoes
1	large or 2 medium onions
1	large clove garlic
2	stalks celery, cut small
2	green sweet peppers
4 to 6	sprigs fresh parsley, Italian preferably
2	tablespoons fresh sweet basil or 1 teaspoon dried pepper and salt
¼	cup dry white wine (optional)

1. Cube the eggplant and slice the zucchini into ½-inch slices, leaving both unpeeled. Slice and cut the onion into small pieces and the green peppers into strips about 1 inch by ½ inch. Mince the garlic. Cut the celery into small, ½-inch pieces.

2. In a good-sized heavy pot heat 2 tablespoons of oil over a medium flame, and then add about one-half of the eggplant, zucchini, and onions. Stir, and allow some to "yellow" or turn light brown; there is not enough oil to brown them all.

3. Remove the vegetables to a bowl, and repeat the process with the remainder of the eggplant, zucchini, and onions. When this batch has reached the yellow-brown stage, sauté the garlic briefly, to a yellow color.

4. Add the contents of the bowl, along with 2 cups of canned tomato. Don't use all of the liquid unless it is needed to cover the vegetables; you may need to add it as the ratatouille thickens.

5. After about 15 minutes of simmering, stir in the cut up

celery, green pepper, parsley, and basil, and cook another 10 or 15 minutes. If the mixture is dry, add the wine. Season to taste.

To serve cold as an hors d'oeuvre or cold salad, chill, and stir in 2 tablespoons of Garlic-Flavored Wine Vinegar for each 2 cups of ratatouille. Sprinkle on additional minced fresh parsley if you like.

This appetizer can also be served hot with a main course at dinner. If Parmesan cheese is grated over it, or a few cheddar cheese cubes are incorporated, it can even be a main dish, accompanied by a salad. Or put ⅓ of a cup of cottage cheese between 2 layers of the ratatouille.

• *Ratatouille Italienne* •

Add to approximately 2 cups of cold ratatouille, one can of flat anchovies from which you've drained off about half the oil. Cut the skinny anchovies in half, stir them in with the remaining half of the oil and 2 tablespoons of Garlic-Flavored Wine Vinegar, and pepper to taste. You won't need salt, since the anchovies are salty enough.

Granted, the basic ratatouille is a bit of a bother, but it has a lot to offer. We often double the basic recipe and serve it hot the day of cooking, and then cold for the hors d'oeuvre.

• *Poor Man's Caviar* •

This simple and delicious cold eggplant dish comes from the Middle East.

1	large eggplant, about 1½ pounds
2	tablespoons oil
1 or 2	cloves garlic
	juice of 1 lemon or lime
2	tablespoons parsley
	pepper and salt
1	small or medium onion, sautéed (optional)
½	cup yogurt (optional)

1. Place the eggplant on a foil-lined baking sheet in a 350° oven for about an hour or until the eggplant is soft to the

touch. Cut it open, let the liquid drain off if it is bitter, or use it if it's not. Scrape the flesh out with a spoon.

2. In a blender, food processor, or by hand with a fork, render the pulp smooth, meanwhile adding the oil, minced garlic, and lemon juice.

3. When the mixture is well blended and free of lumps, stir in the parsley, pepper, and salt.

This is sometimes eaten with hot or cold sliced sautéed onions on top, or with cold yogurt.

• Dilly Beans •

      1 pound firm green beans, as uniform in size as possible
    ½ cup white vinegar
      2 tablespoons sugar
2 or 3 sprigs fresh or dried dill weed, or 1 tablespoon dill seed
      1 teaspoon each salt, mustard seed, and whole black peppercorns
      2 medium onions, sliced
      2 cloves garlic

1. Steam the whole beans for about 10 minutes, drain, and reserve the liquid.

2. Simmer ¾ cup of the bean liquid with the vinegar, sugar, and seasonings. Then add beans, onions, garlic, and let simmer another 10 minutes. Allow the beans to cool in the liquid.

3. Divide the beans in two pint jars with a sprig or so of dill, or the seeds, and one of the garlic cloves in each. Try to get the beans standing up in one direction, in a little bundle.

Serve after three days. This will keep in the refrigerator up to two or three weeks.

• Raw Vegetable Appetizers •

Almost everyone knows and uses cold cut up vegetables, but there are a few things to note. Select a wide variety if you're having a large number of people, but if you're preparing this for only a few, select one vegetable such as cauliflower or broccoli whose remainders you can use for a meal the same or the next day.

Include the usual celery and carrot sticks and small tomatoes, but also really fresh string beans, cucumber sticks, red and green pepper, and radishes. Raw sliced mushrooms of top quality are a lovely addition, as are scallions. Some more unusual choices are julienned strips of white turnips, zucchini, or parboiled celery root. Be fanciful in the arrangement, contrasting the form and colors. Frame the vegetables with a bed of watercress or deep green lettuce.

• *Herbed Cottage Cheese* •

This is not a dip, though it comes close in consistency.

1   pound cottage cheese, regular or low-fat
½   cup scallions or 2 tablespoons grated onion
Optional are any, or all, of the following:
1½   tablespoons celery seed or minced dill weed or chives
½   cup diced red or green pepper, celery, radishes, or cucumber
    pepper and salt

Fold the scallions and any other ingredients into the cottage cheese, season to taste, and let stand for about an hour in the refrigerator before serving.

• *Stuffed Cold Vegetables* •

Use the Herbed Cottage Cheese, or some variation of it, to stuff celery stalks, midget tomatoes, or quartered green peppers.

1. Select medium-sized celery stalks, saving the larger outside ones for cooking. Trim the bottom but leave some of the green tops on.

2. Use a small knife or grapefruit spoon to scoop out some of the pulp of the tomato, which can be used in another way.

Fill the tomato carefully with the cottage cheese mix, but don't pack too firmly. Use a little paprika for color if you haven't any green pepper in the mix.

• *Dips* •

Try these instead of the usual sour cream dips.

Basic combination:
- ½ cup mayonnaise
- 2 tablespoons chili sauce or ketchup
- ¾ cup yogurt

Gradually stir the chili sauce or ketchup into the mayonnaise. When this is blended, fold in the yogurt and whatever set of seasonings you like.

Option 1: Add 1 teaspoon dry mustard, 2 tablespoons grated onion, ½ teaspoon ground pepper, 1 teaspoon Garlic-Flavored Wine Vinegar, pepper, and salt.

Option 2: Add 1 tablespoon grated horseradish, 1 minced garlic clove, 1 tablespoon lemon juice, ½ teaspoon ground pepper, dash of salt.

Option 3: Add 2 tablespoons curry powder, ½ teaspoon ground cumin, 1 teaspoon grated onion, ½ teaspoon ground pepper, dash of salt.

Option 4: Improvise.

CHAPTER 19

Soups

SOUPS ARE the unsung nutritional standbys, waiting and ready to be crammed with nutrients. They can be a satisfying and delicious substitute for an otherwise fatty and rich main course. At least once a week, try to serve a main meal of soup, an expanded salad, bread, fruit, and beverage. This low-fat, high nutrient menu will go a long way toward helping you meet your Dietary Goals.

The choices in soup preparation vary from powdered, dehydrated Something or Other in a Cup, with a pharmacopoeia of ingredients, all unrecognizable except for the noodles, to some idealized country-kitchen soup pot simmering for days, its nutrients lost through overcooking.

Canned soup has its place on the emergency shelf and can be nutritionally perked up with vegetable broth instead of water, thin slices of carrots, and for taste, a teaspoon of wine or whatever's on hand. Condensed chicken broth, especially, is a mainstay among canned foods.

For real soup, try one of your own making. It's a process that gives you so much leeway that a soup recipe is almost a contradiction. Still, we'll offer some basic combinations and a few guidelines. Many of the following soups require assembling rather than long cooking, some can be put together with the help of canned broth, and only a few need an hour or so of slow simmering. But all will be *yours*, not Mr. Campbell's or Mr. Heinz's, and the taste and food value will reflect that.

Soup Know-How

Almost any soup benefits from a very small amount of something acid. We keep a bottle in the refrigerator into which leftover wine is poured. We don't mix red and white in the same bottle because there are times when you don't want a red color. If you have no open wine and you do have a dry sherry or vermouth available, use only half the amount that you would of wine, and taste in a few minutes. Good wine vinegar or a squeeze of lemon can also be used.

Tomatoes: Canned (or frozen tomatoes if you grow your own) have a good amount of liquid that is just the right consistency for a number of soups. Neither tomato juice nor the much heavier puréed, sauce-style tomatoes will do for soups. If you grow and freeze your own, you know there's a lot of excess liquid, even with plum tomatoes. We freeze some of this simply as tomato broth, and it's ready to have on hand when needed. It's also a fresh addition to canned tomato juice, lightening the sometimes too heavy consistency.

Seasonings: Salt, as little as possible, and pepper are basics. Bay leaf, fresh dill, and Italian flat parsley are invaluable. Another good seasoning is dried imported mushrooms which, unlike the fresh, should be given at least one-half hour of cooking time.

Avoid seasoned garlic and onion salt. The fresh versions are easy to keep and use, the flavor is superior, there are no additives, and sodium intake is not increased because of a need for garlic or onion flavor.

Blending: One of the great inventions of all time is the comparatively inexpensive blender. The blender (or food processor) is invaluable for thickening a soup, to liquefy one of the ingredients, to mix in all kinds of bits.

Blend a vegetable instead of using a roux, or flour-and-butter-based thickening, or an egg-and-cream thickening, which some recipes call for. Take a cooked potato or carrot, or whatever is in the soup, add a small amount of liquid, and whir in the blender; then return to the pot and stir in. The amount of potato or other vegetable will be in proportion to the quantity of liquid.

Other thickeners, particularly for hearty soups, include just about all the cereal family: oatmeal, barley, rice, cracked wheat (or Wheatena), and, for a very delicate soup, if you have it on hand, farina.

Browning vegetables is a technique known to every cuisine less meat-consuming than ours. It is particularly helpful when you have no chicken stock available or wish your soup to be austerely vegetarian without it tasting so. Put just enough Garlic-Flavored Oil in a soup pot to cover the bottom. After it is well heated through, put in the cut up vegetables you intend to use — carrots, onions, and so on — and sauté until yellow, not brown. More delicate ones such as mushrooms should only be added for the last minute or two. Proceed from there.

There are several types of soups, from elegant bouillon to thick, hearty concoctions. We lean to almost-stews or to "cream" (without cream or flour) soups because they are more nutritious and hearty enough to satisfy the appetite.

A primary law is simply that water dilutes nutrients and flavor. Hence the proportion of water to your basic soup element must be carefully assessed. If it's too little, you've got gravy; if too much, dishwater. To avoid this, many soups start with a broth (really a stock) that is one step removed from water. Chicken broth is a most versatile liquid to have on hand, in the refrigerator or freezer, either your own or canned. We generally avoid beef-based stocks.

There are two easy ways to produce a homemade low-fat stock from which you can make dozens of soups. The first involves a chicken you can use in the same meal, or later.

• *Chicken Stock #1* •

1	2½–3 pound chicken, fryer or broiler
1 or 2	packages extra chicken giblets (optional). If not included, diminish water by 1 cup.
2½	quarts cold water
1	bay leaf
1	large onion

3   stalks celery, uncut
1   carrot, peeled or scrubbed clean, uncut
6   sprigs parsley

1. Rinse the whole chicken and giblets, removing pin feathers and any fat that can be pulled off. Put it in a large pot with the onion, bay leaf, and cold water.

2. If you use the giblets, let them simmer for about 20 minutes before you add the whole chicken.

3. When the chicken has simmered about 35 minutes, add the remaining ingredients. Let simmer another 35 minutes and test for doneness by cutting into the leg joint. If there is no pink liquid, the broth is done.

4. Discard the onions, parsley, and bay leaf. Let the pot cool without removing the chicken and vegetables.

Later, put the stock in wide-necked jars, from which the fat can easily be removed. Place the chicken, celery, and carrots in a separate dish. The chicken can be reheated along with the vegetables, dill, and some cooked noodles, or with brown rice for a kind of Chicken in the Pot. It can also be used for a casserole or cold for elegant sandwiches. It will have more food value and flavor than an older and fatter fowl, which would require 2½ to 3 hours of cooking. Conversely, the stock will have a slightly less rich flavor, which we think is an acceptable swap.

• Chicken Stock #2 •

3–4   pounds giblets and/or necks and backs
      other ingredients from Chicken Stock #1

Follow the procedure given for Chicken Stock #1, but let the broth simmer for one and a quarter hours.

After cooling, remove the giblets, and discard the tough parts as well as the skin of the necks and backs. Cut off the flesh from the bones, and with the gizzards, whir in the blender or food processor for a minute or two. (The blender may need to have this amount divided into two loads.) The resulting paste can be used cold as a sandwich filling (add a little chopped onion, celery, pepper, mayonnaise, and lemon juice) or put back to thicken the broth. Pour the stock into wide-mouthed jars and store when cooled in the refrigerator or freezer. Remove all fat when the broth is chilled.

• Chicken Stock #3 •

Campbell's Chicken Broth, undiluted. Keep a can or two in the refrigerator, but before using, lift the blob of fat off and discard it. Unlike the homemade stocks, this is salted, so little or no added salt should be required when this is used in soup.

• Turkey Stock •

After roasting and eating a turkey, especially a good-sized one, use the carcass for stock. The proportions below are for a 12 to 15 pound bird.

  All available turkey bones, broken at the joints
2 onions
2 celery stalks
2 carrots
2 bay leaves
  About 2–2½ quarts water, or part (up to one-third) liquid from canned tomatoes, not tomato juice, or other mild vegetable broth

1. Barely cover all ingredients with water or broth. Let simmer for about an hour to an hour and a half, covered. Keep the flame low or you'll end up with only a cup or two of broth.

2. If you plan to use the stock immediately, add any leftover turkey gravy, cut up giblets, or a can of chicken broth for the last 15 minutes of cooking, plus any thickener — cooked rice, barley, dried peas, or noodles. Or ¼ cup of these can be put in, raw, about three-quarters of an hour before you intend to serve.

• Vegetable Stock •

There is seldom need to cook a vegetable stock ahead of time if you save all vegetable liquids; store them in a jar in the freezer or refrigerator. In the case of "strong" vegetables be judicious.

• Legume Stock •

Whenever you cook dried legumes, unless you are simply starting a pot of soup, there should be some extra liquid. Save whatever you have in the same manner as the vegetable stock.

Legume-based soups are old favorites for soup makers. From lentil and split pea to more exotic black bean, they usually share a common denominator: "Take a ham bone . . ." Well, it's not necessary to have a nitrate-laden smoked meat to season dried beans. Here's how.

• Basic Lentil or Split Pea Soup •
Serves 4

1	cup dried peas or lentils
1	tablespoon oil
1	large onion, cut up
1	carrot, cut up
1	large celery stalk, sliced
1	bay leaf
1	clove garlic, minced
3½	cups water
2	cups tomato broth or part vegetable broth
1	can chicken broth, undiluted
	pepper

1. Rinse the peas or lentils, discarding those that float to the top or look unusual, and put them aside.

2. In the soup pot heat the oil and sauté over a medium

flame all the vegetables plus the bay leaf, adding the garlic when the others have yellowed.

3. Empty all of this into a bowl and reserve.

4. Put the washed peas or lentils in the same pot along with the water and cook them for about 35 minutes. Add the broth and vegetables, cook for another 25 minutes until all are tender, and serve hot.

The variations are innumerable: Add diced raw potatoes, oatmeal, any green vegetable, or whatever leftovers you have on hand. Flavor can be changed by adding more tomatoes or a teaspoon or so of curry and a dash of turmeric.

• *A Different Bean Soup* •
Serves 3 or 4

¾   cup navy or other white beans, soaked if necessary
3   cups water
1   tablespoon oil
1   large onion, chopped
1   bay leaf
1   clove garlic
2   cups chicken broth
    salt and pepper
    minced parsley

1. Sauté the onion and bay leaf in the heated oil, and when yellow add the garlic. Cook another minute or so, and then add the washed and sorted beans and the water.

2. Let simmer until the beans are tender, perhaps an hour and a half, depending on the variety of bean. It may be necessary to add water from time to time to keep the beans covered.

3. When they are tender, add the chicken broth and simmer another 10 minutes. Remove the bay leaf, season to taste, and whir in the blender. Two loads may be necessary. If the soup is too thick, add more chicken broth.

Serve with minced parsley.

Variation: For a quick and easy soup, start with cooked

beans, add some sautéed onion and garlic, and then simply blend with the broth and simmer for a few minutes.

• More-or-Less Minestrone •
Serves 5 or 6

Some soups provide two courses. This one is made without the fatty ham and the rather large amount of oil usually called for.

1½–2	tablespoons oil
2	medium onions and 1 cup each of cut up celery and carrots, sliced cabbage, and spinach (or just about any other vegetable you have handy)
1	clove garlic, minced
1	bay leaf
½	cup pink or red beans (cranberry or kidney; presoak if needed)
4	cups water or part vegetable broth
1	frying chicken, whole or cut up
1	can beef broth
1	cup drained tomatoes, or cut up fresh
1	cup tomato liquid
1	teaspoon dried sweet basil or 6 leaves fresh
4	sprigs parsley

1. In a large pot sauté vegetables (except cabbage and spinach) in hot oil until they are yellow, then add garlic and bay leaf. Reserve.

2. In the same pot simmer the beans in the water or vegetable broth for about 20 minutes.

3. Add chicken, broth, tomato, and tomato liquid, and let simmer about half an hour.

4. Add the sliced spinach or cabbage, sautéed vegetables, basil, parsley, and bay leaf, and simmer another half-hour.

You can serve the chicken as a separate course after the soup or cut up pieces and serve all together.

Any number of substitutions and additions can be made. Try adding ½ cup of small cut pasta or some cooked cereal for the last 10 minutes of cooking.

• *Hearty Cabbage and Beet Soup* •
Serves 5 or 6

This is another two-course soup, good to do the day before you plan to serve it, since after chilling the fat and bones can be removed.

1	pound lean chuck
1–2	pounds beef bones
2	onions, sliced
1	large clove garlic, minced
1	bay leaf
4	cups water
2	cups canned tomatoes, at least half liquid
2	cups chicken broth
⅓	head cabbage, about 3 cups, including outside leaves
	pepper and salt
3	canned, sliced beets, with ¼ cup liquid (or fresh if available)

1. Combine beef, bones, onion, garlic, and bay leaf, and all liquids except that from the beets, and simmer until meat is almost tender.

2. Add thin-sliced cabbage and cook over a low flame for another 20 minutes.

3. Add beets for an additional 5 minutes and season. Soup is ready to serve, either with the meat as a separate course or in one bowl.

An almost required accompaniment, if the soup is to be a meal in one dish, is a bowl of steaming hot, thin-skinned potatoes, with minced dill and yogurt as a side dish. Season to taste.

• *Nothing-in-the-House Soup* •
Serves 2 or 3

2	teaspoons oil
1	large carrot, sliced

1   celery stalk, sliced
1   medium onion, sliced
1   potato, sliced
2   cans chicken broth
½   cup tomato liquid
    pepper

1. Heat the oil and sauté carrot, celery, and onion until yellow.

2. Add the potato, chicken broth, and tomato liquid. Let simmer until all the vegetables are tender.

This can be served as is, or some of the vegetables can be blended for thickening.

• *Mushroom and Watercress Soup* •
Serves 4

This recipe method can also be used for broccoli, zucchini, or summer squash soup, and is almost as quick cooking. If you use cooked broccoli, substitute part of the liquid for broth.

1   tablespoon margarine
⅓   pound mushrooms
1   large onion, sliced thin
1   cup watercress or 2 cups green escarole or romaine
         lettuce
3   cups chicken broth
1 or 2   tablespoons white wine or substitute
         pepper

1. In a medium-sized pot heat margarine and sauté mushrooms and onion until yellow.

2. Add greens, broth, and water. Let simmer another 5 minutes.

3. Remove ½ cup or more of the vegetables and whir in blender. Return to pot, add wine and pepper to taste, simmer another 5 minutes, and serve.

• *Winter Squash or Pumpkin Soup* •
Serves 4

2   cups cooked winter squash
3   cups chicken broth
1   small onion, cut up
1   tablespoon white wine
½   cup milk (optional)

1. Prepare the squash by baking at 375° until tender or use leftover unsweetened squash.

2. Purée the cooked squash in a blender with the onion and some of the chicken broth.

3. Return the mixture to the pot with the remainder of the broth and wine. Simmer for 10 minutes.

4. If the soup needs thinning, slowly add milk but do not allow it to boil. Serve with a sprinkling of chives or sliced scallions.

Almost any soup recipe calling for a cream sauce can be converted by using a larger proportion of vegetables to be puréed, some chicken broth, and adding 2 percent fat or skim milk in somewhat smaller quantity than the whole milk called for. Two examples follow.

• *"Cream" of Tomato Soup* •
Serves 4

2½   cups canned or fresh tomatoes
1   large potato, peeled and cut up small
1   onion, cut up
1   stalk celery, cut up
1½   cups or 1 can chicken broth
¾   cup tomato liquid
1   bay leaf
1 to 2   cups 2 percent fat milk

1. Simmer tomatoes, potato, onion, and celery in the chicken broth and tomato liquid until all are tender.

2. Transfer to the blender and purée in one or two loads.

3. Return to the pot, add bay leaf, and add milk until the desired consistency is reached. Taste for seasoning and, if you wish, add a teaspoon of margarine. Serve hot or cold.

• *Spinach Soup* •
Serves 3 or 4

1	potato, peeled and cut up
2½	cups chicken broth
1	cup cooked spinach or ½ pound raw
1	small onion, sliced
½	cup milk

1. Simmer the potato in the broth until tender (with the spinach if raw is being used).

2. Purée the potato, onion, and cooked spinach.

3. Return the purée to the pot, slowly adding milk until the desired consistency is reached. Let simmer for a few minutes before serving. Serve hot or cold.

• *Gazpacho* •
Serves 4 or 5

4	medium tomatoes
1	cucumber, peeled and cut up
1	onion, sliced
1	green pepper, seeded and cut up
1	clove garlic, cut up
3	cups tomato juice
1	cup tomato liquid
2	tablespoons wine vinegar
1	tablespoon oil
⅛	teaspoon cayenne pepper (optional)
	salt to taste

1. Combine the first five ingredients with 1 cup of tomato juice and whir in blender until puréed. Stir in the remaining juice and canned tomato liquid.

2. Stir in the oil, vinegar, and seasonings.

3. Chill it very well for at least 4 hours, and serve with cut up scallion, green pepper, and perhaps toasted whole wheat croutons.

4. If the consistency is too thick, add more tomato juice or serve over an ice cube.

CHAPTER 20

Main Dishes

THE GOAL in main-dish cooking is to supply an important percentage of the day's nutrients and to satisfy the need to feel truly well fed, while avoiding the overindulgence in fats and proteins that are usually associated with this part of our diet.

Here are some suggestions to help you reach this goal:

1. Reduce the size of your meat, poultry, or fish portions to no more than four ounces, preferably three. A scale is a big help here, but you can soon learn to estimate accurately by dividing the weight of a package of meat into servings and using that size as a guide. These portions, which are the standard used by the Department of Agriculture for calculating nutrients in food, are going to look *very* small at first. Make up for the lost quantity of meat with extra vegetables or the starchy complex carbohydrates that are so lacking in our diet.

2. Establish a weekly main-meal pattern in which you eat poultry two times a week, meat two times, and fish once. For the remaining meals, try a hearty soup and salad combination, a pasta dish, a bean casserole, or an egg dish.

3. Buy meat with several meals in mind. If you buy a pound of chopped beef for four people, take out a heaping tablespoon, wrap it well, and stow it in the freezer. You won't miss it. With bits of well-wrapped meat pieces in your freezer, you'll always have the makings of an easy, inexpensive combination main dish on hand.

You can also use this principle of putting aside small portions of meat with cooked food. A roast or broiled chicken can boost the next day's main meal if you cut off a leg or thigh before you serve it. Dice it up the next day into a chef's salad or a Chinese brown rice dish.

4. Learn to think of meat less as an individual dish and more as a part of another dish. Serve spaghetti with a thick meat sauce instead of meatballs, to get all the protein you need and plenty of taste for half the amount of meat. (Make the sauce the day before and skim off the fat before reheating it.) Instead of a cholesterol-rich piece of beef or calf's liver, use a few chicken livers in a sauce to dress up rice or pasta. Although chicken liver is as high in cholesterol as beef liver, it is lower in fat and calories, and a little bit goes a long way.

5. When you are adapting a main dish recipe, cut down drastically on the amount of butter or fat; you won't taste the difference.

6. Where two eggs are called for to bind other ingredients, substitute 2 tablespoons of skim milk or an egg white for one of them.

7. Sauté onions and celery in a small amount of oil and add them to mixed dishes and casseroles to give them a meaty taste or to enhance a small amount of meat. Do as the French do: mince onions, celery, carrots, garlic, mushrooms, and green pepper; sauté them quickly in oil, however, not butter, and add them to almost anything.

8. Use your imagination with seasonings to replace the excessive salt and fat. Grow your own fresh herbs. Experiment with dried herbs and spices — cautiously, but with courage. Each has its devoted users somewhere in the world, and one may strike your palate equally right. Seeds — from popular sesame to tiny poppy — are a high-nutrient addition to main dishes, especially where grains and legumes are included. Buy the seeds in a busy natural food store to be sure they're fresh, and buy them in small quantities since they tend to get rancid. See page 99 to learn more about herbs and spices.

9. Cook one batch of legumes or grains for two or three

meals. One serving can be as a main dish the day you make it, one for a soup, and one for a snack or lunch, all from the original simmering pot that doesn't even require watching.

Here are seven days of main course suggestions that may balance old tastes with newly recognized nutritional needs. Add bread and a simple dessert to complete the meal. All the recipes will be found in this and other chapters in Part III.

Day 1. Bean or lentil soup and a chef's salad with cheese cubes.

Day 2. Spaghetti with meat sauce, marinated cold broccoli and carrot sticks.

Day 3. Broiled chicken, brown rice, peas, waldorf or tossed salad.

Day 4. Chicken minestrone and a salad plate of cold beets vinaigrette with cottage cheese.

Day 5. Kidney bean casserole, cole slaw, and raw vegetables.

Day 6. Eggplant Parmesan, baked potato, and bean salad.

Day 7. Brown rice and fish casserole, cooked spinach or other green vegetable, and tossed salad.

Poultry Main Dishes

• *Lemon Broiled Chicken* •
Serves 4 or 5

2½–3 pound split or cut up fryer or broiling chicken
        juice of 1 lemon (or substitute ¼ cup dry white wine)
    2 slices onion, grated or squeezed in a garlic press
    1 tablespoon Garlic-Flavored Oil
        pepper and salt

1. Rinse the chicken quickly, wipe dry, and remove all pieces of fat.

2. Combine the lemon juice or wine, grated onion, oil, and pepper and salt.

3. Rub the marinade into the chicken, and try to get some between the skin and the flesh. Allow to stand for at least a half-hour.

4. Preheat oven to broil, and meanwhile place the chicken skin side up on a rack on top of a foil-lined broiling pan. Reserve the remaining lemon juice marinade.

5. Place the pan about three or four inches from the heating element, and when the chicken has browned sufficiently, turn it over and baste with the reserved marinade, not the pan juices. If both sides are brown but there is still a bit of pink at the joint when cut into with a knife, turn the oven down and allow the chicken to bake for about 10 minutes at 375°. The whole process should not take more than 35 to 40 minutes for a split chicken, less for one cut in pieces.

6. Lift the chicken from the pan liquids and serve it on a hot platter. Later, carefully scrape up all the bits and pieces from the broiling pan and save all the liquid. When this cools discard the fat that rises to the top and treasure the jellied essence that remains, either in the refrigerator or freezer. It is invaluable for flavoring casseroles, soups, and mixed dishes of all kinds.

• *Roast Chicken* •
Serves 4

Select a good-sized fryer or broiler of about three pounds rather than a roasting chicken which is considerably fatter than the younger broiler-fryers. Rinse the chicken quickly, wipe it dry, and remove any pieces of fat.

1   3-pound chicken
1   tablespoon Garlic-Flavored Oil
    pepper and salt
1   onion
1   celery stalk
    a few sprigs parsley
1   bay leaf
2   tablespoons white wine or lemon juice

1. Rub the chicken with the oil, pepper, and salt, and place breast side down on a V-shaped rack in a small open roasting pan. Put the onion, celery stalk, parsley, and bay leaf in the cavity. Place in oven preheated to 400°.

2. After about a half-hour turn the chicken breast-side up. Continue to roast for another 40 minutes, basting with a little wine or lemon juice. Check for doneness by inserting a thin knife in the leg-thigh joint. If the juice runs clear it is done.

Save the pan juices, as with the previous chicken recipe.

• *Cantonese Chicken with Green Pepper* •
Serves 2 or 3

This is a very useful basic recipe. Try the variations that follow.

 1 whole raw chicken breast, about 12 ounces, cut up in 1-inch pieces
 1 clove garlic, minced
 1 tablespoon soy sauce
 1 teaspoon cornstarch
    pepper
 2 tablespoons oil
3–4 green peppers, cut in strips
 6 scallions, including some of the green part, cut into 1-inch lengths
 3 celery stalks, cut in ½-inch pieces
 1 large onion, sliced
 ½ cup chicken broth
 1 tablespoon cornstarch
 1 tablespoon dry sherry

1. Mix the first six ingredients together and let them stand for about 20 minutes.

2. Heat one tablespoon oil and sauté the peppers, scallions, celery, and onion for about 2 or 3 minutes, stirring meanwhile. Remove from the pan to a bowl.

3. Heat the remaining oil, drain the chicken, reserving the marinade, and sauté the chicken until it has turned color.

4. Add the vegetables to the chicken in the frying pan and stir-fry for about 8 to 10 minutes.

5. Combine the broth, reserved marinade, tablespoon of cornstarch, and dry sherry, and stir this mixture into the

chicken and vegetable mixture until it is well heated through.

Serve this dish with rice, steamed green beans, or broccoli sprinkled with minced scallions.

Variations: Add raw tomatoes, or lightly sautéed mushrooms, at the last few minutes. To heighten the seasoning add a slice of fresh ginger root, minced, or 1 teaspoon of dry ginger. Or substitute spinach, broccoli, or green beans for the green pepper.

This dish can also be made with razor-thin slices of beef or pork instead of chicken.

• *Turkeyburgers* •
Serves 4 or 5

Ground turkey is a new addition to some supermarkets, particularly in the Midwest and parts of the East Coast. Ground fresh turkey, a mix of dark and white meat, is sold in packages similar to ground beef. We have found it a very useful meat — somewhat dryer than hamburger with considerably less fat — but it does need a little flavor-boosting.

1	pound ground turkey
1	small onion, grated
2	tablespoons minced parsley
2	tablespoons dry skim milk
¼	cup tomato liquid (juice or from canned tomato or broth)
	pepper and salt
3	teaspoons Garlic-Flavored Oil
¼	cup bread or cracker crumbs

1. Combine all the ingredients except the oil and crumbs, and form into flat patties.

2. Pat them with one teaspoon of oil, then sprinkle the bread crumbs over the patties, pressing in with your hands if necessary.

3. Heat the remaining oil in a frying pan and sauté the

patties until crisp and brown. These are better well done than rare.

Variation: These can be broiled also.

• *Curried Turkey with Spinach* •
Serves 4

1½	tablespoons oil
1	medium onion, sliced
1	large clove garlic, minced
1	teaspoon fresh ginger, minced, or 1 teaspoon powdered
2	tomatoes, cut in chunks
1	teaspoon curry powder
1	teaspoon turmeric
4	tablespoons chicken broth
¾	pound ground turkey
	salt and pepper
10	ounces to 1 pound fresh spinach, washed, chopped, and dried (Do not use frozen spinach as it gives off too much liquid.)

1. In a large skillet heat the oil and fry the onion until it yellows.

2. Add garlic, ginger, and tomatoes for a minute or two, then the turmeric, broth, and curry powder.

3. Add the turkey, pepper, and salt, and cook for an additional 5 minutes, stirring occasionally.

4. Add the spinach, cover, and cook until the spinach is done, about 5 to 8 minutes. Stir two or three times.

Serve over cooked brown rice.

Meat Main Dishes

• *Quick and Easy Chili* •
Serves 6 or 8

Although there is less fat and less beef, this recipe has more flavor than a typical chili dish.

1	pound chopped beef
1	tablespoon sunflower oil

2 green peppers, seeded and cut in about ½- or 1-inch
   squares
3 large onions, cut small
3 cloves garlic, minced
3 tablespoons chili powder
1 large bay leaf
1 tablespoon cumin, ground
1 tablespoon oregano
1 large can tomatoes (28 ounces)
   pepper and salt
2 cans pinto or kidney beans, size 2½ or 3

1. Cook the meat in a large, heavy-bottomed pot, stirring until no red shows. Drain off and discard all the fat and put the meat aside.

2. In the same pot heat the oil and sauté the peppers and onions until the latter are yellow. Add the garlic, chili powder, bay leaf, oregano, and cumin. Stir and cook for another 2 minutes.

3. Add the tomatoes, breaking up any large pieces, then the meat. Cover the pot and let it simmer for an hour. Stir occasionally.

4. Empty the two cans of beans, liquid and all, into the meat and tomato mixture, and continue cooking for another 25 minutes or so. If the chili seems too dry add more liquid: tomato broth, chicken broth, or part wine. If it is too soupy, simmer uncovered for the last 25 minutes. The amounts of spices are for a moderately hot chili; add less or more chili powder and cumin according to your taste. Of course, this dish can be made with beans soaked and cooked at home, but it is one of the logical places to use canned beans, since the amount of seasoning masks the subtlety of the bean flavor.

• *Hungarian Goulash* •
Serves 4 or 5

A little meat goes a long way in this recipe because of the rich-tasting gravy, served over rice or noodles.

1½–2 tablespoons oil
2 large onions, sliced
2 green peppers, sliced
1 clove garlic, minced
1 pound lean boneless beef (or part well-trimmed pork or veal shoulder) in 1-inch cubes
1 bay leaf
2 tablespoons paprika, Hungarian if available
½ teaspoon sweet marjoram
1½ cups canned tomatoes with liquid
¼ cup dry wine, red or white
1 teaspoon caraway seeds
pepper and salt

1. In a large, heavy pan heat half the oil and sauté the onions and green peppers until the onions are yellow. Add the garlic and cook another minute, then remove the vegetables and set aside.

2. Heat the remaining oil in the same pan and sauté the meat cubes and bay leaf.

3. When the meat is lightly browned drain off the remaining oil, add the paprika, marjoram, and tomatoes and let simmer, covered, for an hour, or until the meat is almost tender.

4. Add the wine, green peppers and onion, and the caraway seeds. Let simmer an additional 15 minutes, and serve over hot cooked noodles or brown rice.

• *Beef with Bean Sprouts* •
Serves 4 or 5

¾–1 pound flank steak, sliced very thin*
1½ tablespoons oil
2 large onions, sliced
1 green pepper, seeded and cut into strips
1 clove garlic, minced

* An easy way to cut meat razor-thin is to partially freeze it to the point of firmness. It then slices perfectly.

1   teaspoon cornstarch
¼   cup chicken broth
1   fresh tomato (optional)
1–2 teaspoons minced ginger root or ½ teaspoon pow-
      dered ginger (or more to taste)
1   tablespoon sherry
1   cup bean sprouts

1. Sear the meat in the hot oil in a large frying pan.

2. Add the onions, green pepper, and garlic, stirring meanwhile, and cook for about 5 minutes.

3. In a small bowl, combine the cornstarch and the broth, and add along with the remainder of the ingredients to the frying pan. Cook for about 5 minutes or more over medium heat. Don't allow the vegetables to become limp. Serve over hot rice.

• *Meat Loaf* •
Serves 4 or 5

Meat loaf is a lovely dish and, with the current cost of beef, certainly can't be looked down upon as plebeian. When you want a decidedly beefy meal this is a good choice because the fat drains off and can be discarded. The oatmeal, skim milk, and wheat germ add nutrition and bulk without sacrificing flavor.

1   pound chopped chuck or round
1   small onion, grated
⅓   cup oatmeal
2   tablespoons dry skim milk
2   tablespoons wheat germ
¼   cup celery, minced
¼   cup green pepper, minced
2   tablespoons parsley
½   cup liquid: tomato or other vegetable broth, preferably
1   teaspoon prepared mustard
2   tablespoons ketchup (optional)

1. Combine all the ingredients except ketchup and mix well. Shape into a loaf and place on the rack of a roasting pan in a preheated 350° oven for about an hour.

2. Spread the ketchup on top halfway through baking.

3. Remove the meat loaf from pan drippings and serve hot or cold.

Save the pan liquid, scraping up all the bits that stick to the pan. Remove the fat when it has chilled, and use the remaining essence as a beef flavoring.

• *Pork Lo Mein* •
Serves 4

½–¾   pound pork, cut in slivers (see footnote at Beef with Bean Sprouts)
1   teaspoon oil
½   cup scallions, sliced
1   clove garlic, minced
1   cup bean sprouts or cabbage, cut fine
1   tablespoon sherry
2   teaspoons cornstarch (optional)
1   cup chicken broth
    pepper and salt
½   pound fine noodles, cooked

1. Heat the oil in a large frying pan and brown the pork quickly, stirring meanwhile.

2. Add all the ingredients except cornstarch and noodles, but reserve a few scallions.

3. Let simmer for about 10 minutes. If thickening is wanted, reserve a few tablespoons of chicken broth, stir in the cornstarch, and add to the pan.

4. Mix in the noodles and heat through. Sprinkle with the remaining scallions, minced fine, and serve in dishes that can accommodate the soupy liquid. Any green vegetable, but especially broccoli and spinach, go well with this. Top with toasted sesame seeds for a good contrast to the noodles.

• Lamb with Green Beans à la Grecque •
Serves 3 or 4

¾   pound boneless lean lamb, cut up, or 1½ pounds lamb
     with bone, in pieces
1   tablespoon oil
2   onions, rough sliced
1   clove garlic, minced
1   cup canned tomatoes, with liquid
1   cup chicken broth
1   pound string beans
¼   cup dry white wine
    pepper and salt to taste
½–1 teaspoon oregano
3   tablespoons flat parsley, minced
4   potatoes, peeled if old, cut in chunks (optional)

1. In a large, heavy pot, sauté lamb in the hot oil, along
with the onions and then the garlic. Drain off all the fat
when the meat is browned.

2. Add the tomatoes and broth, and simmer for about a
half-hour.

3. Add the string beans, wine, pepper, salt, oregano, and
parsley. If potatoes are used they should be added now, with
some extra broth. Turn the mixture occasionally so that uncooked portions will be under the liquid. Cook another 30
minutes after vegetables are added, or until they are tender.

• New York–Style Stuffed Cabbage •

1   3-pound cabbage
½   cup uncooked white rice or 2 cups cooked brown rice
1   medium onion, minced
½–¾ cup lean hamburger meat
1   large clove garlic, minced
     salt and pepper
1½   tablespoons brown sugar
1   bay leaf
2½   cups canned tomatoes, partly liquid

½ cup canned undiluted beef broth
2 or 3 thin lemon slices
2 tablespoons raisins (optional)

A large, deep kettle of boiling water is needed for this.

1. Place the cabbage in the kettle long enough to allow the leaves to wilt, so they can be removed without breaking. Using tongs and a sharp, small knife, cut off the leaves at the base of the cabbage until you reach the core. There should be 15 to 20 usable and limp leaves (small tears don't matter). Cut out the large ribs of the leaves, stack them up, and put them aside with the torn bits for later.

2. In a bowl combine the rice, onion, meat, garlic, pepper, and salt. Divide the meat and rice mix into as many portions as there are leaves, and place one on each leaf. Wrap the leaves around the mix, envelope-style.

3. Cut the remaining cabbage into thin slices, place in the empty pot, and add the beef broth and canned tomatoes, cut up somewhat. Stir in the sugar, bay leaf, and lemon slices, and heat to a boil.

4. Place the cabbage envelopes, seam side down, carefully on the tomato and cabbage mix. Cover and reheat. Let simmer for about an hour. The cabbage should be done but not soggy.

5. If raisins are used, add them in the last 10 minutes.

Egg Main Dishes

• Supper Omelet for Two •

2 eggs
4–6 ounces Egg Beaters or other egg substitute
2 teaspoons water
pepper and salt
1½ tablespoons margarine

1. Combine all the ingredients except the margarine and beat lightly.

2. Heat the margarine until it is bubbly in a nine- or ten-inch frying pan over a medium-high flame.

3. Pour the egg mixture in, tilting the pan and lifting the eggs with a fork until they begin to set. The bottom should be golden, not brown, and the top soft.

4. When it is done fold the omelet over onto hot dinner plates, not a serving plate. If possible, whatever hot food is accompanying the omelet should be on the plate. An easy baked potato, topped with chives, goes well.

Variations: Have sautéed mushrooms ready to place on the omelet before folding; or a mixture of tomato, green peppers, and onion simmered for 5 minutes or so.

• *Farmer's Omelet* •
Serves 2

1	medium onion
2	boiled potatoes (leftovers are fine)
½	green pepper (optional)
2	tablespoons margarine
2	eggs
4–6	ounces Egg Beaters or other egg substitute
	pepper and salt

1. Slice the onion and potatoes, and cube the green pepper, if used.

2. In a large frying pan heat the margarine and sauté the onion, potatoes, and pepper until yellow-brown.

3. Beat the eggs, Egg Beaters, and seasonings together vigorously, and pour over the onion and potato mixture, tilting the pan to allow the eggs to set. Maintain a low to medium flame until the eggs are firm to your taste.

Do not attempt to turn or fold this omelet.

• *Italian Spinach Casserole* •
Serves 4 or 5

1	tablespoon oil
½	cup chopped onion
1	clove garlic, minced or squeezed
1	package frozen spinach

½ cup wheat germ
½ teaspoon dried sweet basil or 2 teaspoons fresh, minced
1 pinch oregano
1 teaspoon parsley, minced
3 eggs
   pepper and salt
4–6 ounces Egg Beaters or other egg substitute
½ cup tomato sauce
2 tablespoons grated Parmesan cheese

1. In a large frying pan heat the oil and sauté the onion, then the garlic, until they are yellow.

2. Chop the spinach leaves and add to the pan. Let the spinach cook until it is soft. Remove to a large bowl.

3. Combine all the other ingredients except the tomato sauce and cheese, and gently stir them into the bowl with the spinach.

4. Pour into a greased 9-inch square or round baking dish. Pour the tomato sauce on top and sprinkle on the grated cheese. Bake in a preheated 375° oven for about 20 minutes.

This is not only an excellent supper dish; cut into small squares it is a good hot appetizer.

· *Egg, Cottage Cheese, and Spinach Bake* ·
Serves 2

This is a lighter, more spinachy version of the previous recipe.

1 package frozen spinach
1 cup low-fat cottage cheese
1 egg, beaten
2 ounces Egg Beaters or other egg substitute
2 tablespoons grated onion
   pepper and salt
1 tablespoon grated Parmesan cheese
2 tablespoons bread crumbs, or part wheat germ

1. Cook the spinach in its own liquid until it is tender and free of juice.

2. Combine the cottage cheese, egg, Egg Beaters, grated onion, and seasonings, mix well, and add to the spinach.

3. Place in a greased shallow casserole or 8-inch pie pan. Sprinkle the cheese and bread crumbs on top, and bake in a preheated 375° oven for about 15 minutes. If a knife inserted in the middle comes out fairly dry, it is done.

Legume Main Dishes

• *Mediterranean White Bean Dish* •
Serves 4

1½ cups dried white beans
1   tablespoon oil
2   large onions, sliced
1   large clove garlic, minced, or 2 small cloves
1   bay leaf
1   fresh tomato, cut up, or 1 canned, drained, and cut up
2   tablespoons tomato paste (optional)
    pepper and salt
2   tablespoons parsley, Italian preferably

1. Place the beans in a large pot, preferably not aluminum, and cover with about a quart of water. Either let soak overnight or bring to a boil for 2 minutes and let soak for 1 hour.

2. Using the same water, though more may be needed to cover the beans by about 2 inches, let simmer for about 40 minutes, or until they are tender.

3. Meanwhile, sauté the onions, garlic, and bay leaf in the heated oil until soft.

4. Add the tomato. Cook until a kind of sauce is formed, about 10 minutes.

5. Add the beans and as much cooking water as needed to make the dish moist but not soupy.

6. Simmer another 15 minutes, and serve with minced parsley on top.

To be truly Near Eastern, accompany this with a bulgur salad and sliced tomatoes and onions.

• Chick Peas and Potatoes •
Serves 2 or 3

This is another Near Eastern combination.

4   small potatoes
1½ tablespoons oil
2   onions, sliced
2   cups cooked chick peas
1   clove garlic, minced
1   cup chicken broth, or more if needed
3   tablespoons parsley or other herbs, minced
    pepper and salt

1. Boil the potatoes (skin on if they are new) in just enough water to cover until they are *almost* tender, slice them and put aside.
2. Meanwhile, sauté the onion until yellow, then add the cooked chick peas and garlic, stirring for a minute or two.
3. Add the broth, salt, and pepper. Add the potatoes to the beans and broth, mix gently, and simmer until the potatoes become tender. Serve with a sprinkling of fresh herbs — dill, parsley, or basil.

• Hopping John •
Serves 4

An adaptation of a typically American southern dish — without the hunk of fatback or lard.

1¼ cups washed black-eyed peas
1   tablespoon oil
1   minced raw onion
¼   cup minced celery
    hot pepper, dry or liquid sauce, and salt
1½ cups *cooked* brown rice

1. Soak washed peas for about eight hours in 6 cups of water. In the same water simmer them until they are tender, about 50 minutes, adding more water if necessary.

2. Meanwhile, in a small frying pan, sauté the onion and celery, and add them to the peas when they are done.

3. Add the hot pepper and salt, and then fold in the rice. Heat through and serve.

Pickle relish is a good accompaniment.

• Dal, or Curried Lentils •

Lentils are a favorite in many lands, but they are a staple in parts of India.

1	tablespoon oil
1	onion, sliced
1	large clove garlic, minced
1	teaspoon fresh ginger, minced, or ½ teaspoon dry ginger
1	bay leaf
1½	tablespoons curry powder
1	teaspoon turmeric
1	cup canned tomatoes, with liquid
	salt and pepper
1½	cups lentils (reddish ones would be authentic, but the familiar brown ones are fine)
	water, about 3 cups

1. Heat the oil in the pot in which the lentils will be cooked.

2. Sauté the onion until yellow, then add the garlic, ginger, bay leaf, curry, and turmeric. Cook for a minute or two and add the tomatoes, breaking up any large pieces and blending in the spices.

3. Add the lentils and water, and let simmer until they are tender. More water may be needed.

Serve this with cut up scallions and cold yogurt.

Other Nonmeat Main Dishes

• *Eggplant Casserole* •
Serves 4 or 5

A most useful, if not outstandingly nutritious, vegetable is the eggplant — but then everything can't be five star. Here it is combined with highly nourishing cottage cheese. The customary first step of frying in quantities of oil is bypassed.

1	1½-pound eggplant
1½	tablespoons oil
1	cup low-fat cottage cheese
½–¾	cup tomato sauce
3	tablespoons flat parsley, minced
1	tablespoon fresh basil or 1 teaspoon dry
1	large clove garlic, minced
	pepper and salt
2	tablespoons grated Parmesan cheese

1. Peel the eggplant in alternate strips, trim ends, and cut in ⅜-inch slices. Sprinkle a foil-wrapped broiling pan with a little oil, place the eggplant slices on this, and dribble the remaining oil over them.

2. Broil under a preheated flame until the slices are slightly brown. Turn and repeat the browning on the other side.

3. In a greased casserole, layer the eggplant, cottage cheese, and tomato sauce, stirring in the parsley, sweet basil, and minced garlic. Top with the grated cheese and bake for about 35 to 40 minutes (or until the eggplant seems tender) in a 375° oven. Cover the casserole for the first 20 minutes and then remove the top.

• *Squash Casserole* •
Serves 4

This is a delicious adaptation of a sour cream and egg-rich recipe.

    4   medium yellow squash (zucchini can be used)
    3   tablespoons cheddar cheese, grated or cut small
    ½   cup low-fat cottage cheese
  3–4   ounces Egg Beaters or other egg substitute
    ¼   cup bread crumbs
    ¼   cup wheat germ
    2   tablespoons minced parsley
    1   small onion, grated
    1   tablespoon Garlic-Flavored Oil
        pepper and salt

1. Grate the squash and let stand in a colander for about 20 minutes. Use the liquid for soup.

2. Mix the pulp with all the remaining ingredients except the oil.

3. Place in a greased casserole, and dribble oil over the top. Bake at 375° for about 50 minutes.

Variation: Reserve 1 teaspoon each of the crumbs and grated cheese to sprinkle on top with the oil.

• *Albanian Vegetable Casserole* •
Serves 3, or 4 if optional vegetables are used

    4   potatoes, sliced thin but unpeeled if new
    2   tomatoes, cut in chunks
    2   carrots, roughly grated
    1   large onion, sliced
    ¼   cup chopped celery
    1   clove garlic, minced
    2   tablespoons parsley
        pepper
    1   can chicken broth
    1   tablespoon margarine
        Optional vegetables: thin-sliced string beans, squash, or peas

1. Place ⅔ of the potatoes in a 2-quart or larger greased casserole. Mix the other vegetables, pour them over the potatoes, and top with the remaining potatoes.

2. Add the chicken broth and pepper, cover, and bake at 375° for about 40 minutes. Uncover, add the margarine to the top, and bake for another 15 minutes. Additional broth may be needed.

Very nice served with a chef's salad.

• *Pasta Al Fresco* •
Serves 4

Spaghetti doesn't have to have a long-simmering, thick sauce. This is light, almost noncooking, and delicious.

<table>
<tr><td>10</td><td>ounces spaghetti or linguini</td></tr>
<tr><td>5</td><td>or 6 quarts boiling salted water</td></tr>
<tr><td>3</td><td>large raw tomatoes, at room temperature, cut up small</td></tr>
<tr><td>1</td><td>tablespoon lemon juice</td></tr>
<tr><td>1</td><td>tablespoon Garlic-Flavored Oil</td></tr>
<tr><td></td><td>pepper and salt</td></tr>
<tr><td>2</td><td>tablespoons Parmesan cheese</td></tr>
<tr><td></td><td>sweet basil to taste</td></tr>
<tr><td></td><td>Italian parsley to taste</td></tr>
</table>

1. Cook the pasta until tender but not soggy. Drain off the cooking water. Do not rinse the cooked pasta under running water.

2. Add the remaining ingredients, maintaining a very low flame for a minute or two while you gently turn the mixture. Serve immediately, preferably in the pot in which you cooked it.

Variations: Substitute 6 or 8 cut up scallions for the tomatoes, or use both; or ½ cup cottage cheese; or 1 cup cooked white beans. For the two latter variations add more pepper and some grated garlic.

Rice

Cooked rice, hot and cold, can be the base for dozens of dishes in many different styles. Even the preparation of plain, unvarnished rice varies from country to country. We recommend these two basic methods as the best for conserving nutrition and flavor.

• Basic Cooked Rice •

Brown rice: Sauté 1 cup of rice in a teaspoon of heated Garlic-Flavored Oil in a heavy saucepan. Stir for a few minutes until the rice changes color very slightly. Meanwhile, have a kettle of water boiling. Take the rice off the flame for a few minutes to avoid splattering, and slowly pour 2¼ cups of boiling water over the rice. Add a pinch of salt, cover, and let cook on a low flame for 45 to 50 minutes. Don't lift the top until a few minutes before that time. Some brown rice requires a bit more water, which you can add then rather than risk having too much liquid. The rice is done when all the water is absorbed and the top has a pitted look. This is true for white rice as well.

White rice: Use converted, the best of the white rices. In a heavy pan place one cup of rice and 2¼ cups of boiling water, plus a pinch of salt and a teaspoon of Garlic-Flavored Oil. Cover and let cook on a low flame for about 18 to 20 minutes.

Variations for both kinds of rice include using seasoned water, vegetable or chicken broth. Interesting additions can be incorporated during the cooking stage or after. We prefer the additions to be made when the rice is done, or almost so, since the flavor is then not diluted by the liquid. Everything from leftover vegetables to chicken, meat, or fish bits, or cheese can be added. Herbs and spices are only limited by your taste.

Here are two rice dishes that are a little more structured.

• Oriental Unfried Rice •
Serves 4

Here's how to have the taste of fried rice without a large amount of oil.

> rice
¾–1   cup chicken broth
  2   tablespoons soy sauce
  ½   cup scallions, cut small
  ¼   cup leftover chicken or pork, shredded
  ½   cup frozen peas, undefrosted
  1   clove garlic, minced

1. Cook either brown or white rice according to the Basic Rice recipe, but using only 1½ cups of water for the white and 2 cups for the brown. Cook for three-quarters of the time suggested.

2. Add all the other ingredients, gently stirring them in. Cover and cook over a low flame another 10 minutes for the white rice and 20 to 25 minutes for the brown.

• *Rice with Mushrooms and Livers* •
Serves 2

A little bit of liver goes a long way in this dish — a good compromise for a food that is rich in iron and other nutrients but also in cholesterol.

    ½   cup rice, brown or white
2 or 3   chicken livers, rinsed and cut up
    1   cup mushrooms, cleaned and sliced
    ½   cup onions, sliced
    2   tablespoons parsley, minced
  ¾–1   cup chicken broth
        pepper and salt

1. Follow the technique in the previous recipe for partially cooking the rice.

2. Meanwhile, sauté the onions, mushrooms, and chicken livers until the onions are yellow.

3. When the rice is three-quarters done, stir in all the remaining ingredients, cover, and complete the cooking.

A variation in preparing this kind of dish is to complete the cooking in a 375° oven, or to do both steps in the oven.

For any such recipe, particularly rice with mushrooms,

you can use bulgur (cracked wheat) as well. This requires only 20 minutes cooking and the same amount of hot water as rice. An excellent food and easy to prepare.

• *Curried Rice with Fish* •
Serves 4

1	cup yogurt
½	cup chopped onions
1	teaspoon turmeric
1	teaspoon curry powder
1	teaspoon ground coriander (optional)
¾–1	pound boneless fish
3	cups Basic Cooked Rice, brown or white
	pepper and salt
1	tablespoon oil

1. Marinate the fish in the first five ingredients for 1 hour.
2. Remove the fish from the marinade.
3. Put the fish on a foil-covered shallow pan under a pre-heated broiler until fish turns color.
4. Mix half the rice with half the marinade and place in a greased casserole.
5. Place the fish on the rice and add the remaining rice and marinade and salt and pepper. Dribble oil over the top, cover, and bake for about half an hour at 375° (longer if the rice is cold).
6. Uncover the dish halfway through baking.
Serve with lemon wedges.
Variation: Use a can of water-packed tuna instead of broiling the fish, and continue with the recipe.

CHAPTER 21

Vegetables

FROM THE MINUTE a vegetable is picked, cut, or dug from its plant the process of vitamin and mineral loss begins. Where it is most accelerated, however, is in cooking, since nutrients are lost primarily through water and heat. Eating vegetables raw is one way to get the maximum in vitamins and minerals, but correct cooking procedures will guard against excess losses.

Water cooking: There are some vegetables to which it isn't necessary to add water. Spinach and other leafy greens, certainly tomatoes, require no additional water; only a watchful eye, medium heat, and, like all vegetable cooking, a pot with a tight-fitting lid.

For those vegetables (potatoes, beets, asparagus, and others) where water is used in greater amounts, the liquid can often be saved for soups and sauces.

As to the amount of heat: don't overcook, and try to time things so that "holding" is minimized. Remember the perils of the institutional steam table, where every bit of nutrition and taste are wafted away as the minutes and hours pass.

Baking is an excellent method for more vegetables than we often realize. Potatoes, white and sweet, are obviously good bakers, but beets, carrots, and summer and winter squash also do well in the oven. And since baking involves a longer use of energy, plan a full utilization of the oven; not only several vegetables, but a fruit dessert or casserole can be baked simultaneously.

Sautéing, or frying in a minimum of fat, is one of the great culinary methods employed by the Chinese and Italians (though we use even less fat than do these cuisines). Almost anything can be sliced thin and sautéed, including a variety of vegetables. Zucchini, string beans, eggplant, celery, and of course potatoes and onions can be pan-fried quickly, alone or in a combination of your choice.

Fry-steam is a very useful variation of sautéing. After light frying, a small amount of liquid is added to the vegetable, such as vegetable or chicken broth, wine or lemon juice, thus creating a built-in sauce so that fattening additions are unnecessary.

Flavor enhancers: Instead of dollops of butter and oodles of cream sauce, experiment with these: lemon juice, onion or onion juice; a teaspoon of margarine combined with lemon, vinegar, or wine; a sprinkling of fresh parsley, dill, or other herb.

For those times when you feel a sauce of some kind is needed, try cottage cheese thinned with skim milk or yogurt and a teaspoon of onion. Whir in a blender and add pepper and salt to taste. Or try the following sauce.

• *White Sauce for Vegetables* •
Makes 1 cup

Skim milk and margarine or oil replace the cholesterol and fat of butter and regular milk. Additional seasonings compensate for their flavor.

    2 tablespoons margarine (or part oil and part marga-
       rine)
 1½ tablespoons white or whole wheat flour
    1 cup skim milk
    1 tablespoon grated onion
       pepper and salt
       Optional: a little grated cheese, fresh herbs, curry pow-
          der, or a little wine or lemon juice

  1. Over a medium flame, using a heavy saucepan, melt the margarine, add the oil, and stir in the flour. Lower the flame

and stir mixture for about 5 minutes. It should not change color.

2. Gradually add the grated onion and milk, continuing to stir another few minutes so that all the milk is incorporated. Add pepper and salt and any optional seasonings.

This will be a medium-thick sauce. Increase the amount of fat and flour to make it thicker; decrease to make it thinner.

Variation: Use vegetable water or chicken broth for the liquid, in which case you might want to add a bit more margarine.

• *Lemon-Flavored Artichokes* •
Serves 4

4	small to medium globe artichokes
4	teaspoons lemon juice
4	teaspoons margarine or Garlic-Flavored Oil
	pepper and salt

1. Prepare the vegetables by cutting off the spiny tips of the outside leaves and all but ½ inch of the stem. Rinse the artichokes and place them in a steamer over boiling water and cook them for about 45 minutes, until an outer leaf pulls off easily.

2. If they are to be served hot, combine the lemon juice, margarine, and seasonings and heat until bubbly. Serve immediately with the lemon juice and margarine in small bowls; pour over or use as a dip. If served cold, allow the artichokes to cool, then press apart the leaves to remove the choke with a sharp teaspoon or knife. Then pour the lemon juice and oil into the heart of the vegetable.

• *Steamed Asparagus* •
Serves 4 to 6

1½–2	pounds asparagus
	lemon juice
	margarine
	toasted whole wheat bread crumbs (optional)

Select stalks of approximately the same thickness. All are equally delicious if fresh and firm, but the thick ones will take longer to cook than the thin ones.

1. Break off the woody ends at the point where they snap. Place the ends in the cooking water while it is reaching the boiling point.

2. If you are cooking less than a pound, use a shallow nonaluminum skillet, and lay the asparagus flat, cover, and allow to simmer for 8 to 10 minutes. If you are cooking a pound or more, cook the spears upright and place them bud side up in the bottom half of a double boiler or other deep pot, in water several inches deep. It helps to tie the asparagus together loosely. Cover and let steam for about 12 minutes, depending on thickness. Save the water and ends for soup, even though some of the ends may be too stringy to eat.

3. Drain the asparagus and serve it on a heated platter with lemon juice, margarine, and bread crumbs.

To serve cold, dress drained asparagus while they are still lukewarm in the same mixture as that used for Lemon-Flavored Artichokes.

• *Green Beans, Creole-Style* •
Serves 4

    1   pound green beans
    1   small onion, sliced
    ½   cup celery, sliced thin
    1   cup tomato, with liquid
    1   bay leaf
         pepper

1. Wash the beans and trim off the ends. Cut them only if the beans are very large.

2. Cook the beans in a steamer until they are half done. Discard the water and place the beans in the bottom of the pot.

3. Combine the other ingredients and stir them into the

beans. Cover and simmer until the beans are tender, about 10 minutes after the tomato mixture has heated through.

• Boiled Beets •
Serves 2 or 3

Beets are sometimes a two-in-one offering. If the bunch you're using has fresh green tops, use the small leaves in salad. The large leaves can be cooked alone or with other greens. This recipe is for the red globes.

6 small beets, about 1 pound
1 teaspoon margarine
¼ teaspoon horseradish
  pepper and salt

1. Cut off the tops to within an inch of the beets, but not the taproot, scrub well and place them in boiling water to barely cover. Simmer until they are tender, about an hour.

2. Lift the beets out, and pour off the liquid carefully so as not to disturb the usually gritty residue on the bottom. Save the water for beet and cabbage soup.

3. Peel the beets by spearing each with a long fork while you slip the skins off with a knife. Return the beets to a small saucepan in which you have a few tablespoons of beet liquid, a little margarine, pepper and salt, and perhaps ¼ teaspoon of horseradish. Beets can also be steamed or baked, covered, in a small amount of water.

• Steamed Broccoli •
Serves 3 to 5, depending on size

1 bunch broccoli
  margarine
  lemon
  pepper and salt

1. Cut off an inch or two of the tough bottom ends of the stalks, place them in water to cover, and cook for about 8 minutes.

2. Put the whole stalks and all available leaves in a steamer over the boiling water for about 8 to 10 minutes. By then the stalk ends in the water as well as the steamed broccoli should be perfectly done. Save the water and ends for soup, serve the leaves and flowering stalks with margarine, lemon, pepper and salt.

• *Quick-Fried Broccoli, Two Ways* •
Serves 3 to 5, according to size

1   bunch broccoli
1   tablespoon oil

1. Slice the tender broccoli stems in ½-inch slices, and, along with the flowerets, sauté them in heated oil for 7 minutes, stirring occasionally.

For a Chinese accent, add 1 teaspoon each of soy sauce, chicken broth, and sherry. Allow the broccoli to reheat, stirring meanwhile, and serve.

For an Italian taste, in the last few minutes add 1 teaspoon of grated Parmesan cheese and pepper and salt to taste. Reheat, stirring, and serve.

• *Brussels Sprouts* •
Serves 3 or 4

1   container (about ¾ pound) Brussels sprouts
    margarine
    lemon juice
    pepper and salt

Steam for about 12 minutes. Dress with margarine and lemon juice, pepper and salt.

• *Cabbage* •

3   cups cabbage, sliced about ¾-inch thick
1   tablespoon margarine
2   tablespoons grated onion

1. Steam for 10 minutes. Remove the steamer and discard the water.

2. In the same pan heat the margarine and the grated onion. Return the cabbage to the pan, heat through, and serve.

An alternate dressing for cabbage is celery, caraway, or toasted sesame seeds, combined with a little margarine.

• Glazed Carrots •
Serves 3 or 4

6 medium whole carrots or 2 cups sliced carrots
1 teaspoon brown sugar
1 teaspoon margarine
1 teaspoon grated orange rind

Carrots may be scrubbed clean or scraped.

1. Cook the carrots in just enough water to keep them from sticking, for about 10 minutes if sliced, for 20 minutes if whole. They should be firm. Do not discard the tablespoon or so of water that remains.

2. Add the other ingredients and heat through, being careful not to let them burn. Serve hot.

The same procedure can be followed for baking the carrots in a hot to moderate oven with a little water in a covered pan.

• Cauliflower •

Cook and serve using the same method as for cabbage, either whole or separated into flowerets.

• Fresh Peas for Two •

Garden fresh peas are among the most cherished of food delights, but, sadly, we usually have to make do with frozen.

1   pound peas
1   teaspoon margarine

Shell peas immediately before using. Steam over water or use a heavy saucepan and a few teaspoons of water. Cooking time in either case should be no more than 10 minutes, and less for fresh picked peas. Dress with margarine. Additions would detract from the special flavor, but you can wrap the raw peas in lettuce leaves before cooking.

• *Potatoes* •

This most maligned of vegetables deserves the kudos it's beginning to get from nutritionists. For variety explore the different kinds available. There is a marked difference in taste and texture between a russet and a thin-skinned potato from California.

It has become automatic, when facing a potato, to reach for the peeler, if not before cooking, then later, thus losing important nutrients. True, with mashed potatoes it is necessary to have skinless pulp, but that's about the only preparation method where this is so. If you're hesitant, try this first dish.

• *Boiled New Potatoes* •
Serves 4

8   small, thin-skinned new potatoes, blemish-free

Scrub potatoes well, put them in water to cover, and let them barely boil for about 15 or 20 minutes, until tender but not overdone. Pour off the water and replace the pan on a very low flame, shaking occasionally so that the potatoes will dry out but not burn. Serve immediately with margarine, pepper, and salt; or cottage cheese; or half yogurt and cottage cheese; or all yogurt; or minced scallion, dill, or parsley.

• *Caramelized Potatoes and Carrots* •
Serves 4

6	new potatoes, fairly large
3	carrots
1	tablespoon oil
1	small onion, grated
4 or 5	tablespoons chicken broth
	pepper

1. Scrub the potatoes and carrots well, and slice in equal widths, about ¼-inch thick.
2. Heat the oil in a large frying pan, and sauté potatoes and carrots and onion over medium heat, allowing them to yellow, not brown.
3. Add chicken broth, cover tightly, and cook for about 10 minutes, shaking the pan occasionally. Add pepper and serve when tender.

• *Mashed Potatoes* •
Serves 4

If you've forgotten how good and how easy-to-prepare real mashed potatoes are, this may be welcome.

6	old potatoes
½–¾	cup skim or low-fat milk
2	tablespoons margarine
1	tablespoon grated onion
	pepper and salt

1. Cook potatoes until they are tender and then peel them (or peel them raw and save the water for soup). Allow potatoes to dry out in the pot over a low flame, shaking occasionally.
2. Using mixing beaters or other method, add all the other ingredients. The right consistency is important, so if you need more milk, this is the time to add it, while maintaining a low flame under the pot. Either serve the potatoes from the

same pot or preheat a greased casserole that you can keep hot.

• Baked Potatoes •

True, you don't need a recipe for this. But please, choose baking potatoes, russets preferably, and scrub the skins well. Don't oil them, and don't put them in aluminum foil. Pierce the skin after they've been in the oven 20 minutes to allow the steam to escape and thus avoid an explosion.

Serve baked potatoes with cottage cheese and scallion or chives, and remember, the skin is good and good for you.

• Spinach and Other Greens •
Serves 3 or 4

The leafy vegetables — turnip and collard greens, kale, swiss chard, beet tops, and the most widely used, spinach — are more popular now that their nutrients and flavor are increasingly appreciated. (The more tender greens are lovely uncooked in salads.)

1. Place 1 pound washed greens in a heavy pot; do not add water. Cover and cook over a low flame. Spinach, swiss chard, and beet greens require only 8 or 10 minutes, while the others may need about twice that.

2. Try adding some minced onion to any green in the last few minutes of cooking time. *After* cooking, cut up the limp strands and dress the greens with either a little margarine or thinned cottage cheese, pepper and salt.

• Summer Squash •

The home gardener's delight and bane, new squash burst forth around mid-season in the minute it takes to retie a tomato plant. But in addition to the summer months, zucchini and yellow squash now appear in the stores with far greater frequency than in prior years, and they are fairly reasonably priced. All of the cooking methods can be used with both, from baking to steaming to sautéing. Summer squash also mix well with onion, tomato, green pepper, and eggplant, either separately or all together, as in a ratatouille (see page 159). And of course when summer squash are really fresh, simply slice them raw for a salad or a snack.

In cooking summer squash there are a few guidelines. Wash the skins with a vegetable brush if they need it but don't peel them. Be aware of the high water content; don't drown or overcook summer squash. If you don't want to serve the liquid given off with the squash, save it for stock.

• Stir-Fry Zucchini •
Serves 4

4   medium zucchini
1½ teaspoons oil
2   tablespoons chicken broth
½   clove garlic, minced or pressed
1   teaspoon or more soy sauce, to taste (optional)
    pepper

1. Slice the washed zucchini into ¼-inch rounds.
2. Heat the oil in a frying pan and add the zucchini, stirring occasionally.
3. When most of the zucchini is yellow add the garlic and chicken broth. Cover and let steam for about 5 minutes until tender but not limp. Add the soy sauce and pepper, stir for a minute more, and serve.

• Broiled Zucchini with Yogurt •
Serves 4

4   medium zucchini
2   tablespoons oil
½   cup yogurt
1   clove garlic, minced or pressed
    pepper and salt

1. Slice the zucchini *lengthwise* in halves, place on a foil-covered broiling pan, and rub well with oil on the cut side of the zucchini and lightly on the skin portions. Place about four or five inches below a preheated broiler and, watching carefully, cook until browned, not burnt.

2. Combine the garlic, pepper and salt, and yogurt, and serve it as a side dish.

• Yellow Summer Squash with Cheese Topping •

Prepare and cook as in the recipe for Broiled Zucchini. Add a few tablespoons of bread crumbs and grated cheese, with or without onion juice, to the squash in the last 5 minutes of broiling.

• Winter Squash •

There are many varieties of winter squash, all highly nutritious (very high in vitamin A and minerals) and very good eating indeed. They are easy to cook but somewhat pesky to prepare. The tough outer skin requires a cutting board and sharp knife. The addition of a mallet makes it easier.

You'll generally find butternut and acorn in the store, but if you see a turban-shaped squash called buttercup, somewhat larger than acorn, grab it. Or if you have a good-sized garden, grow this variety. The deep orange flesh not only signifies more carotene, the vitamin A precursor, but also superb flavor.

• Baked Squash •
Serves 4

2   acorn squash, or 1 butternut, or 1 buttercup
1   tablespoon margarine
1–2 tablespoons brown sugar, maple syrup, or honey

1. Rinse squash and then, using a heavy knife and hammer or mallet, cut into the squash to divide in half. Scoop

out the stringy fiber and seeds. (We save the seeds, letting them dry in the pilot light of the oven and then toasting them when the oven's on. Either we or the birds get to nibble on them.)

2. Place the squash cut side down in a foil-lined flat tin with sides that has about ¼ cup of water in it. Bake at 350° to 375° for about 40 minutes.

3. Turn the squash right side up, testing the *flesh*, not the skin, for softness with a sharp fork. It should be yielding but not mushy. Place a dab of margarine and some of the sweetener in each cavity. Let bake another 15 minutes or until fork-tender. Serve hot.

Variation: Add applesauce or apple juice to the cavity, and a dash of cinnamon or nutmeg.

• *Sweet Potatoes or Yams* •

Yes, the caloric count is comparatively high, but the nutrients are in proportion. They should be enjoyed simply baked in the skin or mashed with a tiny dab of margarine; there is no need to gild this lily with heavy syrup or marshmallows. Select the so-called yams, those with the deep orange flesh.

Wash one potato to a person, bake in a preheated 375° oven for 40 to 45 minutes, or less time at 400°. Pierce with a fork during the last 20 minutes of baking to let the steam escape.

• *Mashed Sweet Potatoes* •
Serves 4

4   sweet potatoes
¼   cup orange juice
1   teaspoon grated orange rind
1   teaspoon sherry (optional)

1. Bake or boil sweet potatoes and peel them when they are tender.

2. Add the other ingredients and mash well, preferably with a mixer.

3. Place in a margarine-greased casserole to reheat. Serve.

• *Broiled or Baked Tomatoes* •

When tomatoes are abundant, or perhaps not of top flavor, you may wish to serve them hot.

4   medium tomatoes
1   tablespoon Garlic-Flavored Oil
2   tablespoons minced parsley
2   tablespoons bread crumbs
    pepper and salt

1. Cut tomatoes in half horizontally and place cut side up on a foil-covered broiling pan. Dribble oil over the cut sides and place four or five inches from a preheated broiler.

2. Broil for about 5 minutes, then sprinkle crumbs, parsley, and seasonings over the tomatoes and continue broiling until they are brown, about another 5 or 10 minutes.

The same ingredients can be baked in a hot oven, for a somewhat longer time.

CHAPTER 22

Salads

SALADS CAN BE what you want them to be: a minor accompaniment or a star performance. Most of the recipes in this chapter are for dishes that are meant to be important parts of our dietary intake.

Since we depend on salad as a means, perhaps the only one, of eating raw vegetables, we should take seriously what goes in the salad bowl. If, for instance, you're having a large wedge of iceberg lettuce, a quarter of tomato, dressed with 2 tablespoons of bottled French dressing, this is how that adds up:

	CALORIES	VITAMIN C	VITAMIN A
Iceberg lettuce	12	5 mg	300 IU
¼ tomato (during the winter)	7	2.5	225
French dressing	132	—	—

The same amount of romaine lettuce, however, has almost twice the amount of vitamin C and ten times the vitamin A of iceberg lettuce. Raw spinach and watercress contrast even more dramatically for vitamin and mineral content with iceberg lettuce. Make sure your choices add up, nutritionally.

Salad, though, is not simply a fine source of vitamins and minerals but is remarkably versatile and easy to prepare. We suggest that salad be a major part of the main meal several times a week. These, naturally, should contain some form of protein and be more substantial than the other kinds.

Salad Guidelines

• Put salad ingredients, unwashed, into the refrigerator as soon as you bring them home from the market.
• Prepare salads as close to eating time as possible, to guard against vitamin and mineral loss. Cut or tear greens shortly before serving.
• Since the outer leaves of greens are the highest in nutrients, discard only those leaves that are actually not usable. If some are a trifle tough simply cut the pieces smaller.
• Wash the uncut vegetables and greens carefully and quickly; don't let them soak in water.
• For salads in which cooked vegetables are used: studies show that cooked broccoli and string beans, among some others, lose considerable amounts of vitamin C after only one day of refrigeration.* (Remember, too, that vitamin C is a kind of barometer of other nutrient losses.) So, handy as it is to prepare several days' supply of cooked food, try to use those leftovers as soon as possible.

Flavor Suggestions

Wheat germ, sautéed for a few minutes in a tiny bit of Garlic-Flavored Oil and allowed to cool, is an excellent addition to a salad.

Toasted sesame seeds offer an interesting contrast to some bland salads, as well as being good nutritionally.

Salad dressing should be light, not heavy; should enhance, not mask, the foods beneath. This usually means a classic oil and vinegar dressing, but there are some combinations such as a red or white cabbage mixture that call for a richer dressing, perhaps the Russian or Thousand Island (yogurt-based) type.

---

*Nutritive Qualities of Fresh Foods and Vegetables, edited by P. L. White and Nancy Selvey, Futura Publishing, 1974.

Oil: Safflower and sunflower oils both have an excellent ratio of polyunsaturates to saturates, and we use them for all cooking purposes *except* salad dressing. Corn oil, with its good but smaller proportion of polyunsaturated fats, is our choice because the flavor is more to our liking. If olive oil is a particular favorite for salad, make sure you use one of the other three in cooking. And try a mix of half olive oil, half corn oil.

Vinegar: Use an unflavored wine vinegar (or cider vinegar if you prefer it); any additions of herbs or seasonings should be made at home. If fresh tarragon is available, a small sprig can be tucked into a vinegar bottle, but we would not want it to flavor all salads. Other herbs, such as sweet basil or dill, are also better added directly to the salad.

Grain and Legume Salads

Salads made with grains and legumes can take the place of the familiar mayonnaise-laden potato, macaroni, and cole slaw salads. They are much more nutritious, some are far easier to prepare, and, with additions, they can be main course dishes as well.

• *Rice Salad* •
Serves 6

3   cups (1 cup uncooked) brown or white rice
2   tablespoons Garlic-Flavored Oil
3   tablespoons Garlic-Flavored Wine Vinegar
½   onion, grated, or 2 tablespoons minced scallion
1–2 tablespoons minced parsley or dill weed

1. Add the other ingredients to the cooked rice, preferably when it is still lukewarm. This adds considerably to the flavor.

2. Add cut up vegetables (cooked or raw), cheese, fish, or chicken bits to make this a main-course dish.

• *Three-Bean Salad* •
Serves 6

3   cups any cooked dry beans or lentils

Follow the same instructions as for Rice Salad, except add a bay leaf and more onion to the beans while you are preparing the dressing.

• *Tabbouleh* •
Serves 5 or 6

1   cup bulgur (or cracked wheat), large cut
2   cups boiling water
1   onion, minced
1½   cups Italian parsley, minced
½   cup fresh mint, if available
¼   cup lemon juice
2   tablespoons oil
      pepper and salt

1. Place the wheat in the boiling water and let it simmer for about 2 minutes.

2. Turn off the flame and let the wheat remain in the water for another 20 minutes or longer, until it has expanded in size.

3. Transfer it to a colander and drain off all the water, pressing it with your hands.

4. Place the wheat in a good-sized bowl, add all the other ingredients, and turn lightly to incorporate the dressing.

Serve with sliced cucumbers, olives, tomatoes, and yogurt.

• *Macaroni Salad* •
Serves 4

8   ounces small macaroni, shells or elbows
2   tablespoons Garlic-Flavored Wine Vinegar
2   tablespoons grated onion

3   tablespoons celery, cut small
2   tablespoons yogurt
2   tablespoons mayonnaise
    pepper and salt

1. Cook the macaroni until it is done but still firm. Drain and let it cool. Shake the strainer or colander to make sure all the water is gone. Sprinkle vinegar over the macaroni and let it stand for at least 10 minutes.

2. Add all the ingredients and blend well. Chopped chives or scallions are a nice topping.

Variation: Instead of the yogurt-mayonnaise dressing, thin ¼ cup low-fat cottage cheese with a tablespoon of mayonnaise and a tablespoon of skim milk. The blender is best for this.

Assorted Vegetable Salads

• *Avocado Salad* •
Serves 6

Avocado is one of the few fruits with a high fat content, so it isn't suitable for concentrated intake. However, keep in mind that those grown in Florida are about 20 percent lower in fat than the California variety. Besides, avocado seems to combine naturally with other, low-fat foods.

2   Florida avocados, peeled and sliced horizontally
2   green or red peppers or tomatoes, sliced equally as
    thick as the avocado
½   cup low-fat cottage cheese
2   tablespoons yogurt or low-fat milk
3   tablespoons mayonnaise
½   cup minced celery
¼   cup minced scallion or grated onion
1   teaspoon horseradish
⅓   cup lemon juice or part Garlic-Flavor Wine Vinegar
    pepper and salt

1. Arrange alternating slices of avocado and green pepper or tomato on a platter.

2. Blend the cottage cheese, yogurt, and mayonnaise. Add the other ingredients until well mixed.

3. Pour the dressing over the vegetables.

• *Broccoli and Lemon Juice* •
Serves 4 to 6

1	large bunch broccoli
4	tablespoons Garlic-Flavored Oil
	juice of ½ lemon, or more to taste
	pepper and salt

1. Cut the bottom stems off the broccoli, leaving the stalks about five or six inches long, and put the tougher stems in the bottom of the pot. Cook about 5 minutes.

2. Place the flowered stalks in the steamer, cover, and let simmer for about 10 minutes, or until barely tender.

3. Combine the oil, lemon juice, pepper, and salt.

4. When the broccoli is done, drain the water and remove the stalks carefully to a serving plate.

5. While still warm pour the dressing over the stalks. Slit them carefully lengthwise to serving-size pieces. Let stand for about a half-hour to cool in the refrigerator, and baste once or twice. Reserve the coarser pieces in the bottom of the pot for soup.

Variation: Add ½ teaspoon of dry mustard to the dressing.

• *Beet Salad* •
Serves 3 or 4

1	pound beets, cooked or canned, sliced
½	cup onion, sliced very thin
1	tablespoon Garlic-Flavored Wine Vinegar
¼	cup yogurt or well blended low-fat cottage cheese
½	teaspoon prepared mustard
1	teaspoon horseradish
	pepper and salt

1. Combine the vinegar, beets, and onion, and set aside.

2. Mix all the other ingredients.

3. Let both stand for about half an hour, and then spoon the sauce over the beets.

• Carrots in French Dressing •
Serves 4

12   whole small or 8 medium carrots, washed and scraped
4   tablespoons French dressing
1   teaspoon dried sweet basil, or 1 tablespoon fresh, or
1   tablespoon fresh mint, minced

1. Steam the carrots or simmer in barely enough water to cover until they are just tender.
2. Pour the dressing over the drained, lukewarm carrots, let marinate for half an hour in the refrigerator, and sprinkle with the herbs. This should not require pepper or salt.

• Basic Cabbage Salad •
Serves 3 or 4

Remember how nutritious those outer leaves are, and stir them in, cut fine, with the lighter ones.

4   cups cabbage, sliced fine and well packed down in the measuring cup
1   onion, grated
2   tablespoons oil
2–3   tablespoons vinegar, to taste
     pepper and salt

Combine all the ingredients and one or more of the following optional additions: shredded carrots, finely diced celery, celery seeds, dill, parsley, or caraway seeds.

• Cabbage Waldorf •
Serves 5 or 6

4   cups cabbage, as in Basic Cabbage Salad
1   large red apple, cut in small cubes

    2   carrots, washed and shredded
    3   tablespoons raisins
    2   tablespoons vinegar, cider preferably
   3–4   tablespoons mayonnaise
   3–4   tablespoons yogurt
         dash of salt

   Combine all the ingredients well. If the slaw seems a little thick, stir in a tablespoon or two of apple juice or milk.

• *German Beet and Cabbage Salad* •
Serves 5 or 6

    4   cups cabbage, as in Basic Cabbage Salad
    3   tablespoons pickle relish or chopped sweet pickles
    2   tablespoons grated or chopped onion
    ½   teaspoon dry mustard, or more to taste
    3   tablespoons oil
    3   tablespoons vinegar
    ½   teaspoon sugar
    1   cup diced apple or boiled potato
    1   cup cooked sliced beets, diced (canned is fine)

   1. Combine the cabbage, relish, and onion.
   2. Stir the mustard into the vinegar to dissolve, and then add all the remaining ingredients, except the beets. Stir well.
   3. Shortly before serving fold in the beets.
   Dill is a good garnish.

• *Fruit Cole Slaw* •
Serves 5 or 6

A variation of an old Midwest favorite.

    4   cups cabbage, as in Basic Cabbage Salad
    1   cup diced canned pineapple, unsweetened, or
    2   oranges cut up, or half and half
    ½   cup raisins

2   tablespoons pineapple or orange juice
3   tablespoons mayonnaise
3   tablespoons yogurt
    salt

1. Combine the cabbage, fruit, and raisins, and mix well.
2. Stir the fruit juice into the mayonnaise until it is absorbed, and then fold in the yogurt and a dash of salt.
3. Combine with the cabbage and fruit mixture.
Variation: a few chopped walnuts sprinkled on top, or some cut up dates incorporated with the cabbage and fruit.

• *Cauliflower with Sesame Seeds* •
Serves 4 or 5

1   small head cauliflower, whole, blanched or raw
2   tablespoons lemon juice
2   tablespoons oil
    pepper and salt
    toasted sesame seeds

1. Wash the cauliflower and dip it in water for a few minutes (look for bugs).
2. Steam the cauliflower for only 5 to 7 minutes unless you're having it raw.
3. Steamed or raw, break the cauliflower into flowerets, and dress with the oil and lemon, pepper, and salt. Serve at room temperature, sprinkled with toasted sesame seeds.

• *Eggplant Salad* •
Serves 3 or 4

1   1-pound eggplant
½   tablespoon oil
1   medium onion, sliced
1   garlic clove, minced
2   tablespoons tomato sauce or 1 tablespoon tomato
    paste
1   tablespoon oil

1　tablespoon vinegar
2　tablespoons toasted sesame seeds

1. Bake the eggplant on a foil-covered broiling pan for about one hour at 375° or until the skin wrinkles and the eggplant seems soft.
2. Meanwhile, sauté the onions, and then the garlic, in the ½ tablespoon of oil until they are yellow but not brown.
3. When the eggplant is done peel the skin off and place the pulp in a large bowl. It will give off a good amount of liquid. If this is bitter, discard it.
4. Blend the eggplant until it is barely puréed but not soupy. If your blender requires liquid for this, either mash the eggplant by hand or add the oil and vinegar at this point.
5. Return the eggplant to the bowl, and by hand mix in all the other ingredients except the seeds. Chill well for at least an hour.
6. Serve on romaine lettuce leaves, sprinkled with the sesame seeds. This is especially good with any kind of Mediterranean meal.

• *German Potato Salad* •
Serves 5 or 6

6–8　potatoes, about 2 pounds, preferably thin-skinned
¼　cup green peppers, thin sliced
1　onion, or 4 scallions, cut up
¼　cup celery, diced, or 1 tablespoon celery seed
3　tablespoons Garlic-Flavored Oil
3　tablespoons Garlic-Flavored Wine Vinegar
　　pepper and salt
1　teaspoon celery seeds

1. Wash the potatoes well, and let simmer until barely tender. Drain and let them cool somewhat.
2. Peel and cube (or slice) the potatoes, and combine with the other ingredients. Turn the salad gently once or twice, distributing the dressing thoroughly. Serve at room temperature. Garnish with dill.

• *American Potato Salad* •
Serves 5 or 6

Follow the recipe for German Potato Salad but substitute: 3 tablespoons mayonnaise, 3 tablespoons yogurt, and 1 teaspoon Garlic-Flavored Wine Vinegar for the oil and vinegar dressing.

In this salad, parsley is preferable to dill. A variation is the addition of 1 tablespoon of pickle relish.

• *Green Beans Vinaigrette* •
Serves 4

```
1   pound green beans
1   large onion, preferably sweet, sliced very thin
4   tablespoons Garlic-Flavored Oil
2   tablespoons Garlic-Flavored Wine Vinegar
    pepper and salt
```

1. Wash and trim but do not cut the green beans. Place in a steamer over boiling water, and cook until they are tender but crisp, about 15 to 18 minutes.

2. Remove them immediately to a large bowl, and while the beans are still warm, add the onions, oil, vinegar, pepper, and salt. Place in the refrigerator to cool until serving time.

Tossed Salads

These are the old reliables, the without-which-it-isn't-dinner for so many of us. Recipes aren't needed, just some general remarks. Remember, when you buy, color counts; the deeper green leafed lettuces have more nutritional value than the pale white heads. Expand your horizons; try combinations new to you. Think small — a whole salad of raw broccoli might be depressing, but a half cup of flowerets among the greens is a welcome contrast.

A while back some of us made a fuss about torn versus cut lettuce. As it happens, there's no difference in nutritive value, certainly none in taste, and the notion that torn lettuce "holds the dressing better" is nonsense. You may prefer one or another method according to convenience or looks.

A tossed salad is generally made up of two or more greens, but there's no reason why one won't do. However, think of additions as nutritive boosts, capable of filling you up as well. The result, then, is

• *Chef's Salad* •

3–4 cups greens, preferably romaine plus some watercress
 ½ small onion, sliced, or 4 scallions, cut up
1¼ cups protein-rich food: diced chicken, diced cheese, cooked chick peas or white beans, or any combination of these
 1 green pepper, diced
 4 tablespoons French dressing
 2 tablespoons wheat germ, sautéed in a little Garlic-Flavored Oil, or whole wheat croutons

1. Just before serving prepare the greens by washing them quickly. Let the water drain off and pat dry.

2. Tear or cut the lettuce into bite-sized pieces and place in a serving bowl.

3. Add the onion, green pepper, and the protein food.

4. If beans are the choice, a little extra pepper and salt can be added to them before combining with the greens.

5. Sprinkle on the dressing and turn several times before adding the wheat germ or croutons, and turn once more.

If good tomatoes are available, slice and serve them as a side dish, rather than incorporated in the salad, to avoid excess sogginess.

• *Spinach and Mushroom Salad* •
Serves 4

Here's another tossed salad, one that has recently become very popular. Our version, of course, does not include the bacon topping that is sometimes added.

1   pound spinach (some other greens can be used in part)
¼   pound mushrooms, best quality, without chemicals
⅓   cup cottage cheese or yogurt-mayonnaise dressing
3   tablespoons garlic-sautéed wheat germ or whole wheat
      croutons

1. Wash the spinach and drain very well; wipe the mushrooms with a damp paper towel. Remove the stems and ribs from the larger spinach leaves, and cut off the stem end of the mushrooms and slice.

2. Combine the spinach and mushrooms.

3. Immediately before serving add the dressing, which can be prepared ahead of time. Toss the salad lightly, and add the wheat germ or croutons.

Cottage Cheese Salads

Old reliable cottage cheese shouldn't be taken for granted. It's good by itself and can incorporate just about anything around, sweet or tangy. Remember that not quite a half cup (100 grams) of 2-percent-fat cottage cheese has 1.93 grams of fat, while the same amount of cheddar cheese has 33.14 grams.

• *Cottage Cheese Platter* •
Serves 2

Combine:

1   cup low-fat or regular cottage cheese
1   tablespoon grated onion
½   cup of one or any combination of diced celery, green
      or red pepper, cucumber, grated carrots, shredded
      cabbage

Dill, parsley, celery, or sesame seeds are always good extras.

• Cottage Cheese Platter •
Serves 4

2   cups cottage cheese
1   cup pickled beets (or sliced tomatoes and cucumbers)
4   lettuce leaves
    any dressing

Divide the cottage cheese between the four lettuce leaves, and place the vegetables around them.

• Cottage Cheese and Fruits •

Almost all fruits seem to go well with cottage cheese; it particularly enhances cooked and canned fruits. Some favorites are apricots, prunes, pineapple, and Elberta peaches.

The best topping, if any is needed, is a teaspoon or two of fruit juice. Or cottage cheese thinned with a little fruit juice or with a teaspoon of honey stirred in.

CHAPTER 23

Desserts

WE CANNOT TELL a lie. Rich, heavy desserts, loaded with sugar and laden with butterfat, will not help you meet your Dietary Goals. Fortunately, there are other ways to pander to your sweet tooth. Fruits and fruit-based dishes make an ideal ending for a meal. Other desserts can simply be de-fanged — adapted so that the maximum of old taste remains, with only a minimum of the old fats and sugars. When adapting recipes, the first guideline is to see where you can make substitutions.

Oil for butter or margarine whenever possible. (However, subtract two tablespoons of oil from a cupful for every cup of solid shortening called for in the recipe.) This can be done in some recipes, including all breads and less delicate cakes. It is not feasible where the recipe calls for creaming the shortening and sugar.

Margarine for butter. We stopped using butter in baking ten years ago with little perceptible taste difference, except to the most super-refined of palates.

Skim milk for whole milk, and dry skim milk both as a replacement and as a nutrient beefer-upper. Add a tablespoon of dry skim milk to every cup of liquid milk.

Yogurt for sour cream. This can be used where sour cream is called for in yeast baking and in pound cake recipes, as well as baking powder coffee cakes. Do, however, heighten the flavorings by an additional half to offset the more acid yogurt flavor. Also, add the yogurt at the very end of the mixing process, since its texture is more delicate than that of cream. If possible, drain off excess water from the yogurt.

Eggs. Compromise is the word here. We keep Egg Beaters on hand, and where a recipe calls for two eggs, we use one plus about three ounces of the substitute, or sometimes double the Egg Beaters and omit the egg.

In some recipes you can substitute egg white for the whole egg. However, if you've internalized the old "waste not want not" maxim, you may have trouble disposing of those egg yolks.

Sugar. Many of the recipes in this chapter contain sugar, often white sugar. The amounts given will be as small as possible to achieve the sweetness desired, which is the point of eating desserts in the first place. The whole array of sweeteners available — honey, maple syrup, cane and beet sugars (both brown and white), molasses — have individual uses. Honey and maple syrup cannot be successfully substituted for sugar in cake, since their texture would disturb the chemistry; white and brown sugar can be interchanged, though the taste will be changed.

Sugar can, however, be cut down in most recipes, even baked goods. One conspicuous sugar saving is effected by eliminating all icings. These are usually a major source of sugar, sometimes even of shortening. Substitute a thin sugar glaze (see page 239) if you must have a topping. Or use a teaspoon of powdered sugar, sprinkled thinly through a paper doily or a sieve.

In evaluating your old recipes, look at the proportions of the ingredients. An acceptable ratio is one cup of sugar to two cups of flour. A recipe that calls for more sugar to flour should be avoided until you experiment by reducing sugar content markedly. We always try to cut down the sugar-to-flour ratio further, sometimes reducing it to three-quarters of a cup of sugar to two cups of flour.

However, conventional cakes — butter, pound, sponge cakes, and their derivatives — are usually heavy in other undesirable ingredients: shortening and/or egg yolks. Two other categories of baked goods, sweet yeast cakes and muf-

fins–tea breads, provide delicious alternatives to the fat-
and egg-rich concoctions of the past.

Yeast Cakes

For a yeast coffee cake recipe yielding two cakes, four cups
of flour requires only a half cup of sugar and a half cup of
shortening for the basic recipe, and perhaps one-quarter cup
additional sugar for a filling or topping. This is also the kind
of dough in which dried and fresh fruit can be easily incorporated.

Yeast baking is sometimes thought of as a cult activity,
difficult and time consuming. It does need to be done when
you're available over a stretch of some hours, but it requires
little more actual work. A rainy day or evening, while you're
occupied with other things, is perfect. And if kneading dough
seems too strenuous, there is an excellent coffee cake that
you can make without your hands touching the dough. Give
that one a try even if you're reluctant to dive into bread
making.

Tea Bread, Muffins, Quick Bread

These easy and versatile baked goods are a fine ending to a
meal. Since everything tastes sweeter when heated, serve
muffins warm. There is little or no difference between the
basic content of recipes, whether given as muffins or loaves,
except in amounts, so you can be flexible in adapting these
from muffin to loaf pans. Adjust the timing — about 55 minutes for the loaf pans and 30 minutes for the muffin tins.

Fresh and Cooked Fruits

The best and most delicious way to end a meal, from the
simplest to the most elaborate, is with fruit. A bowl of even a
single kind of fruit can be perfect if the bowl is your prettiest
and there's an interesting accent for the fruit, a small garnish of dried fruits or nuts.

Timeliness plays a part too. In late October, crisp new McIntosh apples give off a special autumnal rightness that they do not have in April, even though they're available. On the other hand, offering hard to come by, out of season fruits and berries is seldom a sound idea. Maximum flavor and nutrition are gained in eating fruit, as well as other foods, in season.

Dried fruits and nuts are always a welcome contrast to fresh fruits in taste and texture, but certain combinations are most apt. Crisp apples and raisins, with walnuts in the shell to prolong the eating process, are naturals. Peaches and pears seem to take to almonds, while tangerines or any good orange is nicely accompanied by a plate of figs or dates.

Of course a mixed fruit bowl, with a whole array from grapes to pineapple, is always elegant, particularly for a large group of people. Any combination is appropriate.

The other way to present fresh fruit, by cutting it up, offers many variations as well. Again the choice is whether to mix two or more kinds. Most of us have a few combinations we rely on, but it's a good idea to change styles occasionally. Sliced oranges, with simply a teaspoon or so of liqueur, are delicious and have the great virtue of being available in one variety or another all year. Peaches and melons, certainly, can take center stage alone.

Pears are one of the few fruits that do not do well cut up, either alone or in a combination. They turn brown quickly, even when dipped in citric juices to hold back the process. Their delicate flavor is lost, too, in a mélange. Serve them French-style, on a pretty plate, with a knife.

Combinations otherwise can be as varied as the season and your tastes dictate, and adjusted for the amounts needed. For fifteen people in June you can contrive an elaborate watermelon basket with cherries, grapes, and even peaches. But in February, say, with an orange and apple in the refrigerator, you can still produce a good fruit mix. Add a few snippets of cut up dried fruits, or add in smaller amounts some canned fruit. Apricots and pineapple are good fillers along with the apple-orange-banana trio. Almost all fruits are enhanced by some added juice. Try some extra orange juice or syrup from canned fruit; or a few table-spoons of liqueur; or a combination of honey and juice; or apple juice; or sherry. If you're using a melon of any kind, after you've cut out the pieces of fruit, scrape out juice from the rind with a spoon. If the melon is a cantaloupe, you can actually squeeze the juice out of the skin. This is the best liquid of all.

If a few extra strawberries are available, mash them lightly with a fork and add a teaspoon or so of sherry or liqueur.

If you're adding cut up dried fruits such as figs or dates or whole raisins, let them soak in whatever liquid you're adding for about ten minutes or longer.

Important: Do cut fruit you're using only a short time before it goes to the table. The custom of preparing a fruit mixture hours before a meal so that the "flavors can blend" is destructive of food nutrients, particularly vitamin C. Have ready what added liquid or dried fruit is to be used, but wait to cut the fresh.

Some fruits take to cooking or baking, and they are included among the recipes.

Cooked Fruits

• *Ginger Pears in Brandy* •
Serves 6

This is a good dessert for company and can be made in advance.

  6 firm ripe pears, Bosc preferably, peeled
  ½ cup maple syrup or brown sugar
  ⅞ cup water
1–2 tablespoons brandy
  ⅛ teaspoon ginger
  ½ teaspoon grated lemon rind

A small, deep baking dish with a cover is needed, large enough to support the upright pears.

  1. Wash the pears, peel them with a potato peeler, and cut

out the blossom end but not the stem. Place them in the baking dish.

2. Combine the other ingredients and pour over the pears. Cover with a top, or aluminum foil, and bake for about 35 minutes in a preheated 375° oven.

3. Check to see if the fruit is becoming tender. Remove the top, baste with the liquids, and continue baking another 15 minutes or until the pears are easily pierced but not mushy. Serve each with a teaspoon or so of the syrup. Reserve any liquid that is left; it can be used to sweeten another fruit, or as a sauce for a dessert, or to flavor yogurt before freezing.

• *Bananas à l'Orange* •
Serves 4

    4   bananas
        juice of ½ orange
        Optional flavorings: 2 tablespoons rum, 1 tablespoon brown sugar, 2 tablespoons honey, sesame seeds

1. Place the peeled bananas on a foil-wrapped broiling pan with any one of the optional flavorings plus the orange juice poured over.

2. Bake in a preheated 400° oven for 10 to 15 minutes or broil under a preheated broiler. Be watchful if the broiler is used. Serve immediately.

• *Glazed Apple Slices* •
Serves 4

    4   firm apples, cored but unpeeled
    2   tablespoons maple syrup or 1½ tablespoons brown sugar
    1   tablespoon lemon juice
        dash of cinnamon
    2   tablespoons margarine

1. Slice the apples crosswise about ¾-inch thick and place them on a slightly greased foil-wrapped broiling pan.

2. Dot the remaining margarine over the slices along with the other ingredients.

3. If they are to be baked, place in a 400° preheated oven for about 15 minutes; if broiled, place the pan under a pre-heated element until the surface of the apples turns bubbly and a little brown. Watch carefully.

• *Baked Apples* •
Serves 4

Good baking varieties are Northern Spy, Rome Beauty, or Cortland.

    4   apples, cored and with stem end peeled about 1½
          inches down
    2   tablespoons butter
    2   tablespoons brown sugar
        scant teaspoon cinnamon
    3   tablespoons raisins

1. Place the apples, peeled side down, in a baking dish with about 1 inch of water.

2. Cover the dish and bake at 350° for about 35 minutes.

3. Invert the apples, combine the other ingredients, and stuff the cavities.

4. Return to oven, uncovered, and bake for another 20 minutes or until the apples are tender. Baste the apples with the pan liquid, and add water to it if it becomes too syrupy. Serve warm.

• *Sherried Fruits* •
Serves 4 or 5

        1   11-ounce box of mixed dry fruits
        2   thin-skinned navel oranges, unpeeled and sliced
              across about ½-inch thick
        ¾   cup fruit juice or water
        ½   cup sherry
  2 or 3   tablespoons raisins, preferably golden

1. In an 11- or 12-inch shallow glass baking dish spread the mixed fruit and oranges, reserving the apricots, add water to cover, and cover the dish with aluminum foil.

2. Bake in a preheated 375° oven for about 20 minutes. The fruit should be almost soft; if not, return to the oven for a few minutes.

3. Add the liquids, apricots, and raisins and replace in the oven, uncovered, for an additional 20 minutes or until all are completely tender. If the liquid cooks out, add more proportionately of both sherry and juice or water. Serve warm or cold. This can be served several days after it is baked, since the flavor and consistency improve.

• Orange-Marinated Prunes •

"Stewed" dry fruits have mysteriously lost favor and should be recalled. They can be a delicious ending to a meal, and should *never* actually be stewed.

⅔ pound, approximately, large dried prunes
2 slices orange, cut about ½-inch thick
   boiling water
1 quart jar, heat-proof

1. Place the prunes in the jar, with the orange slices at the bottom and middle.

2. Add the boiling water slowly until the prunes are covered. Screw the top on and leave at room temperature for 6 to 8 hours. Refrigerate for several days before using.

Variation: For spiced prunes add a small piece of cinnamon stick and two cloves.

Baked Desserts

• Meringues with Fruit for Eight •

A special-occasion dessert, completely fat free, with very little work.

⅔ cup egg whites (about 4 eggs) at room temperature
1 cup sugar
   pinch of salt
1 teaspoon lemon juice
   strawberries, washed and hulled, or other fruit
   Optional: whipped topping, custard topping, liqueur

1. In the large bowl of an electric mixer beat the egg whites at high speed until they become frothy.

2. Begin adding the sugar slowly until all is beaten in, using a rubber spatula frequently to scrape the sides. The whole process should take about 4 minutes.

3. Add the salt and lemon juice and beat another minute, making sure there is no liquid egg white on the bottom of the bowl.

4. Cut a large, clean brown paper bag to fit two flat cookie tins.

5. Shape the meringue in rounds about 4 or 5 inches across, using a soup spoon and knife, and drop onto the brown paper-lined tins. Swirl the egg white in a circle. (If you wish this can be done with a pastry bag, but we don't think it's worth washing out for this simple task.)

6. Bake at 275° for about 1½ hours. The meringues should barely turn color but be firm enough to slide or be nudged off the paper with a spatula and knife.

7. Test one to see if you can remove it without breaking the meringue. If it is still sticky, return the pans to the oven until they are dry enough to be removed. If some crack, they can be placed together so that the fruit filling covers the split. The recipe provides for a few extra in any case.

Store carefully in a covered tin for as long as three or four days if you wish.

8. At serving time place a meringue on each plate, fill with fruit, and, if no topping is added, mash a few strawberries and combine with some liqueur to incorporate in the fruit.

Variations: Peaches or raspberries, the ultimate luxury, can be used, or, more prosaically, a combination of sliced oranges, bananas, and canned apricots. Sprinkle with liqueur.

• *Two-Layer Cake* •
Serves 8

There are times, such as children's birthdays, when an old-fashioned, simple American layer cake is wanted. The egg substitute and skim milk boost its nutrient quotient.

   2   cups unbleached white flour minus 2 tablespoons
2½   teaspoons baking powder
   ½   teaspoon salt
   1   stick margarine
   1   cup sugar minus 2 tablespoons
   ⅓   cup Egg Beaters or other egg substitute *
   1   egg
   ¾   cup skim milk
   2   tablespoons dry skim milk, diluted in liquid milk
   1   teaspoon vanilla
        All ingredients should be at room temperature.

Grease and flour two 8-inch round pans.

1. Sift the combined flour, baking powder, and salt, and set aside.

2. Cream the sugar and margarine, add the egg and Egg Beaters and beat for 2 minutes at high speed if using an electric mixer, or vigorously by hand.

3. Fold in the dry ingredients by thirds, alternately adding the skim milk and vanilla. Blend well but do not beat after the flour has been added.

4. Pour the batter into two pans and bake on the middle rack of preheated 350° oven for about 35 minutes. The cakes are done when the batter shrinks slightly from the sides of the pan, or a toothpick comes clean when inserted in the middle of the cake.

5. After 10 minutes, remove the cakes from the pans by

---

*In this and all other recipes, an additional egg may be used instead of the substitute.

carefully running a knife around the rim and gently whacking the pan's bottom. Place the cakes on a rack to cool so that the steam given off will not collect and make them soggy.

If an icing is necessary, use a small amount of this one.

ORANGE GLAZE

⅓ cup powdered sugar
    juice of ¼ orange
    grated peel of one orange
 1 teaspoon orange marmalade, optional

Gradually add the juice to the sugar, stirring to smooth the lumps. Add the grated peel and marmalade. This will be somewhat more of a sauce than an icing. Put cake together as layers, or cut into squares when cool.

Variation: Put a few tablespoons of apricot preserves between the layers, and a sifting of confectioners' sugar on the top.

• *Cottage Pudding* •
Serves 4 to 6

Along the lines of the two-layer cake but with even less margarine and fewer eggs is this very old-fashioned baked dessert served warm with fruit.

⅓ cup margarine
⅔ cup sugar
¼ teaspoon salt
 1 egg or ⅓ cup Egg Beaters or other egg substitute
 2 cups flour minus 2 tablespoons
 3 teaspoons baking powder
⅞ cup skim milk
 2 tablespoons dry skim milk
 1 teaspoon vanilla

Follow instructions for the Two-Layer Cake. Our grand-mothers served this warm with a cornstarch lemon or choco-late sauce. A more nutritious topping is the orange glaze in the preceding recipe, in doubled amount, heated slightly. Lightly mashed peaches, strawberries, or other fruit are good too.

• *Orange Tea Bread* •

    2 cups unbleached white flour minus 2 tablespoons (½ cup whole wheat flour can be substituted for the same amount of white flour)
    ¾ cup sugar
    3 tablespoons dry skim milk
  1½ teaspoons baking powder
    ½ teaspoon baking soda
    ¼ teaspoon salt
    ½ teaspoon cinnamon
    ¼ teaspoon allspice
    1 egg or ⅓ cup Egg Beaters or other egg substitute grated rind of 2 oranges
    ½ cup orange juice
    ¼ cup oil
    ½ cup nuts and ¼ cup raisins (optional)

Grease and lightly flour a loaf pan.

1. In a large bowl stir all the dry ingredients well; sifting is not necessary.

2. In a small bowl beat the egg until light, and then stir in the oil, rind, and juice.

3. Add the liquid to the dry mix all at once, and stir in until all the flour is dampened. Add the nuts and raisins if used.

4. Pour into the greased pan and bake for about an hour in oven preheated at 350°. Test for doneness. This will proba-bly crack in the center; tea cakes generally do.

Allow to stand in the pan for about 10 minutes, and then remove and invert on a rack. Do not attempt to cut a tea loaf when it is still hot.

• Bran and Raisin Loaf •

1   cup unbleached white flour
¾   cup whole wheat flour
3   tablespoons wheat germ
3   teaspoons baking powder
½   teaspoon baking soda
1   teaspoon cinnamon
½   teaspoon salt
½   cup brown sugar
1   cup whole bran cereal
¼   cup oil
1   egg or ⅓ cup Egg Beaters or other egg substitute
1½   cups skim milk
3   tablespoons dry skim milk
⅓   cup raisins

Grease and flour a loaf pan.
1. Mix the flours, baking powder, soda, salt, cinnamon, sugar, and wheat germ in a large bowl and set aside.
2. In a small bowl combine the milks, egg, oil, and bran. Stir quickly, and then add to the flour mixture. Stir in the raisins and pour into the loaf pan.
3. Bake in a preheated 350° oven for about 50 minutes. Test for doneness and, if ready, remove from the oven and allow to stand for 10 minutes. Cool loaf, inverted, on a rack.

• Basic Plain Muffins •
Makes 12 to 16 muffins, depending on tin size

1½   cups unbleached white flour (up to half can be whole wheat)
2   tablespoons wheat germ
½   teaspoon salt
2   teaspoons baking powder
½   cup dry skim milk
⅓   cup sugar, brown or white
⅓   cup oil
1   egg or ⅓ cup Egg Beaters or other egg substitute

½ cup water
2 teaspoons grated orange rind
Optional additions:
¼ cup walnuts, cut up
¼ cup raisins
1 cup grated, unpeeled raw apples
4 or 5 prunes or dates, snipped into small pieces
1 teaspoon cinnamon

1. In a large bowl stir together well the flour, wheat germ, salt, baking powder, skim milk, and sugar.

2. In a smaller bowl combine the oil, water, and egg.

3. Mix the liquids quickly, without beating, into the flour mixture.

4. Fill greased muffin cups ⅔ full and bake in oven preheated at 400° for about 20 minutes or until brown. Serve hot.

• *No-Knead Yeast Coffee Cake* •
Makes 2 coffee cakes

This is easy, but you must be in the house during the entire process. You will need an electric mixer to make this cake.

1 package dry yeast (or 1½ packages if you want to hurry the process)
⅓ cup warm to hot water — about 115°
1 teaspoon sugar
1 stick margarine
1 egg
½ cup Egg Beaters or other egg substitute
½ cup white sugar
1 teaspoon salt
1 13-ounce can skim evaporated milk, or 1 cup yogurt plus ¼ cup liquid skim milk
4 cups unbleached white flour
1 cup raisins
2 teaspoons grated orange rind (or part lemon rind)

1. Place the warm water and sugar in a straight-sided 8- or 10-ounce glass. Stir in the yeast and put in a warm place and let rise 5 minutes or so.

2. Meanwhile, gently warm the skim milk or yogurt. Since yeast is a living organism that can be killed by over- or underheating, all these precautions are important.

3. In a large mixing bowl place the margarine, egg, Egg Beaters, sugar, and salt, and pour over the milk or yogurt.

4. Add 2 cups of flour and turn the mixer on low speed only until the flour is incorporated.

5. When the yeast mixture has risen, add it to the large bowl, scraping out all the yeast with a spatula.

6. Start the mixer again, and keep it on low speed for about 4 minutes, using the spatula occasionally to push the dough toward the beaters.

7. After 4 minutes add the grated rind and the raisins and slowly add another cup of flour. Continue to use the mixer while adding flour until the mixture starts to "run" up the beaters.

8. Turn mixer off and add the remaining flour by hand, beating in vigorously with a strong spoon or broad silver knife.

9. Cover the bowl with a damp thin cloth and put in a warmish place; a gas oven with a pilot light is perfect.

10. Let rise until the mixture is light and almost doubled. With one yeast package this will take close to 2 hours.

11. After this first rising beat the dough for a few seconds. Have ready two well-greased loaf pans or any baking tins with high sides. Divide the batter into the two pans. Place the pans in the same warm spot to rise again. They do not need to be covered for this rising, which will only take about ¾ hour.

If your cakes have risen in the oven, leave the pans in and turn the oven to 350° when the dough is ready. If they have risen elsewhere, preheat the oven to 350° and place them gently inside. Bake about 50 minutes to an hour. Remove cakes from the pans immediately by running a knife around the edges. Invert on a rack to cool. If you wish, top with the orange glaze on page 239.

Variation: As you spoon the dough into the baking tins before the second rising, sprinkle a mix of a few spoons of brown sugar, nuts, and ½ teaspoon of cinnamon on one layer of the dough, and then cover with more batter. This gives a cinnamon vein running through the coffee cake.

•   •   •

There is no possible way to put Mom's apple, pumpkin, or lemon meringue pie on the acceptable list, but there is one type of pie that is fine by any standard. You can vary the flavor, as long as you maintain the approximately 1⅔ cup of fruit pulp and liquid to 1 package of gelatin. The reason for a graham cracker crust as opposed to a conventional two-crust, shortening-based one is that it contains about ⅔ less calories and fat. In time, try cutting down on the margarine even further, by reducing it a tablespoon or two.

An alternate egg white crust, sometimes called angel pie or schaum torte, is given after the pie recipe.

• *Apricot Chiffon Pie* •

GRAHAM CRACKER CRUST

¾	cup crushed graham crackers
⅓	cup wheat germ
1½	tablespoons sugar
¼	cup melted margarine

Combine all the ingredients and press with a spoon and fingers into a lightly greased 9-inch pie pan. Bake in pre-heated oven at 350° for 8 to 10 minutes, watching carefully to prevent burning.

FILLING

8 or 10	canned apricots, enough to make ¾ cup purée
1	teaspoon grated lemon rind
⅔	cup apricot liquid
¼	cup water

1 envelope unflavored gelatin
1 tablespoon sugar
1½–3 tablespoons Grand Marnier or other fruit-based liqueur
1 cup low-fat plain yogurt
1 or 2 egg whites (two will make it fluffier)

1. Combine the apricots, gelatin, rind, apricot liquid, sugar, and water in a saucepan, place over low heat, and stir until the gelatin dissolves. Remove from the flame and allow to cool. Stir in the Grand Marnier.

2. Place the mixture in a large bowl and gently fold in the yogurt. (If any liquid has risen to the top of the yogurt, discard it for this recipe.)

3. Chill until the mixture is almost firm, about two hours.

4. Beat the egg whites until they are stiff but not dry, and fold them into the apricot-yogurt mix.

5. Spoon this into the baked, cooled graham cracker crust, and with a knife create a peaked, not smooth, top.

6. Return to the refrigerator to chill another hour before serving.

Variations: For prune chiffon substitute ¾ cup cooked prune pulp for the apricot pulp. Apricot nectar or orange juice may be substituted for the apricot liquid. If orange juice is used, increase the sugar by 1–2 tablespoons. The other ingredients are the same. For strawberry chiffon substitute 1 cup strawberries, most of which should be slightly mashed, and the liquids described in the prune chiffon version.

SCHAUM TORTE CRUST

3 egg whites
¾ cup sugar
½ teaspoon lemon juice

1. Beat the egg whites until they are foamy.

2. Gradually add the sugar until stiff peaks form, and beat another minute. Add lemon juice.

3. Spread in a well-greased 9-inch glass pie pan, building up the sides with a spatula.

4. Place in a pre-heated 275° oven for about 1¾ hours. Check earlier to see that the meringue is drying but not becoming golden.

5. Fill the meringue shell in its glass pan; do not attempt to remove it to serve.

This will not cut into neat slices, but it is delicious.

Cookies

The following three recipes are comparatively high in nutrients and low in fats and sugars. Still, restraint must be practiced, since they are also delicious.

• *Oatmeal Cookies* •
Makes about 75 cookies

1½	sticks margarine
1	cup brown sugar
¼	cup white sugar
1	egg or ⅓ cup Egg Beaters or other egg substitute
¼	cup oil
¼	cup water or apple juice
1	cup unbleached flour
1	teaspoon cinnamon
½	teaspoon allspice
	dash of ginger
3	tablespoons dry skim milk
¼	cup wheat germ
1	teaspoon salt
½	teaspoon soda
3	cups old-fashioned Quaker Oats
½–¾	cup raisins, chopped nuts, or dates in any proportion

1. Beat together the margarine, sugars, and egg until creamy.

2. Stir in oil and water or juice.

3. Mix together the flour, spices, skim milk, wheat germ, salt, and soda, and add to the creamed mixture.

4. Fold in the oatmeal and raisins with another quick beating.

5. Drop by spoonfuls onto a greased cookie tin. Bake for about 15 minutes in oven preheated at 375°, then immediately remove cookies. If you wish to bake only part of the batter and freeze the rest, shape into a roll and wrap. This freezes well for several months.

• *Sherry Cookies* •
Makes about 55 cookies

1¾   cups unbleached white flour
⅓   cup wheat germ
      pinch of salt
½   cup sugar
 1   stick margarine
 1   egg
¼   cup oil
 3   tablespoons sherry
½   cup walnuts

1. Combine the flour, wheat germ, and salt, and set aside.

2. In a large bowl cream the margarine, sugar, and egg, then add the oil and sherry.

3. Add the flour mixture to the large bowl and mix well.

4. Stir in the walnuts.

5. Place spoonfuls on greased cookie tins, and press down to flatten, either with an oiled soup spoon or the fleshy part of your thumb. Bake in preheated oven at 350° for about 12 minutes, remove from the pan, and let cool.

• *Peanut Butter Cookies* •
Makes about 60 cookies

½   cup brown sugar
¼   cup white sugar
½   cup oil

1   egg or ⅓ cup Egg Beaters or other egg substitute
¾   cup peanut butter
¼   teaspoon allspice or ½ teaspoon cinnamon
½   teaspoon salt
1½   cups unbleached flour (or part whole wheat flour)
3   tablespoons wheat germ

1. Combine the first five ingredients and beat on low speed with an electric mixer or by hand.

2. Combine and add allspice or cinnamon, salt, flour, and wheat germ gradually, incorporating it with the hands if necessary.

3. Place 1-inch balls about 2 inches apart on a greased cookie tin, and press them flat with the tines of a fork. Bake in preheated oven at 375° for about 15 minutes, remove, and cool.

• *Brown Edge Cookies* •
Makes about 55 cookies

This is a somewhat less virtuous cookie to serve with fruit.

1   stick margarine
1   cup sugar
1   tablespoon grated orange rind
½   cup orange juice
1   egg or ⅓ cup Egg Beaters or other egg substitute
½   teaspoon cinnamon or ⅛ teaspoon ginger
2   cups unbleached white flour
½   teaspoon baking powder
2   teaspoons dry skim milk

1. Cream together the margarine and sugar and then the egg, rind and juice. Put aside.

2. Combine the flour, baking powder, dry skim milk, and cinnamon or ginger, and mix thoroughly.

3. Add to the creamed mixture, stirring well.

4. Drop by teaspoonfuls on a well-greased cookie tin. Bake in preheated oven at 350° for about 12 minutes or until the cookies are a light brown.

Gelatin Desserts

These are so simple to make it is very hard to understand the lure of Jell-O, Royal, and others with their artificial everything and high sugar content. The basic recipe calls for combining unsweetened, unflavored gelatin with a little less than two cups of the liquid of your choice, from fruit juice to coffee to wine.

• *Apricot Nectar Dessert* •
Serves 4

    1   envelope gelatin
    1   small can apricot nectar
    2   tablespoons water
        juice of one orange
    1   tablespoon lemon juice
    1   tablespoon orange liqueur (optional)

1. In the bowl in which you intend to serve it sprinkle the gelatin into ½ cup of nectar.
2. In a small saucepan heat to a simmer ½ cup of the nectar and the water.
3. Pour the hot mixture over the gelatin, stirring vigorously to dissolve all the grains, and add the remaining nectar, orange and lemon juice, and liqueur if desired. Let chill until firm, about three or four hours.

• *Orange Gelatin* •
Serves 4

    1   envelope unflavored gelatin
    1¾   cups orange juice
    2   tablespoons lemon juice
    ¼   cup sugar
         pinch of salt
         fruit: 1 sliced banana, cut-up apple, or orange

1. Sprinkle the gelatin into ½ cup of the orange juice in a serving bowl.

2. Meanwhile, heat 1 cup of the juice with the sugar and salt until it barely comes to a simmer.

3. Stir it immediately into the gelatin until it is dissolved and there is no trace of grains on the bottom of the bowl.

4. Stir in the additional orange and lemon juice. Let it chill for about an hour or so before you stir in the sliced fruit. Continue to chill until it is firm.

• Whipped Gelatin •

Follow the recipe for Orange Gelatin. When the gelatin is almost jelled, whip with a rotary beater and return to the refrigerator and continue to chill. Fruit can be added at this point if you wish.

• Apple Gelatin •

Follow the Orange Gelatin recipe, substituting apple juice for the orange juice, and subtracting 2 tablespoons sugar. Add sweet grated apple (McIntosh is good) either to the plain or whipped gelatin.

• Coffee Gelatin •

Use medium-strong fresh coffee as the liquid, about 2 tablespoons sugar, and 1 tablespoon rum instead of the lemon. This seems to call for a whipped topping. See page 155.

Frozen Dessert

• Orange Sherbet •

Serves 8 or 10

While this is a nutritious substitute, it does not have the consistency of machine-made sherbet, so it is best frozen in the individual dishes in which it will be served.

1   cup nonfat dry milk
3   cups water
4   tablespoons sugar
1   tablespoon grated orange rind
1   cup orange juice
2   teaspoons lemon juice
½   cup strawberries (optional, but very good)

1. In a large bowl combine the dry milk and water, stirring out the lumps.

2. Add the remaining ingredients except the strawberries. Pour into a loaf pan to freeze until the mixture is almost hard.

3. Remove the sherbet from the freezer and beat well. Stir in the strawberries and return to the freezer. Repeat the process once more for a good texture, though it can be served after the first beating. Pour into individual containers unless you plan on serving it all at one time. It is more difficult to cut into than ice cream. Remove from the freezer about 20 minutes before serving.

CHAPTER 24

Bread

THERE ARE MANY cookbooks devoted entirely to the baking of bread, and even more with excellent chapters on this subject. At least one, *Joy of Cooking* by Irma S. Rombauer and Marion Rombauer Becker, has excellent illustrations of the process. All that we would like to do here is to urge the consideration of bread making as part of your normal routine, not as an exotic essay into the unknown. In this way the bread you eat, just about every day, can be your own, with the assurance that its contents are the best. A freezer is needed if you begin baking in quantity; but whether it's eight loaves or one, a day is required when you can be on hand for a good stretch of time.

The bread mystique is a perplexing phenomenon. People who spend a good deal of time preparing an elaborate dessert that will be eaten in minutes feel they have neither the skill nor the hours to make bread, just about the most satisfying and nourishing of foods.

Because yeast, bread's leavening, consists of living organisms, once activated it requires certain conditions. When these are learned you are in complete mastery of the process and can be as flexible as you wish about the contents, procedure, and even timing. (For instance, dough can be refrigerated at several stages, when you become proficient.)

To begin: The granules in the yeast envelope (cake yeast is harder to work with and is frequently sold stale) have the job of raising the other ingredients. They can do so only if the liquid they combine with is between 105° and 115°. The addition of a small amount of sweetener hastens the process.

Directions on the yeast envelope suggest mixing the dry ingredients, including yeast, and adding a warm liquid to this. The old-fashioned method is to let the yeast rise in a small amount of liquid while you're assembling the dry ingredients. We find this preferable, if for no other reason than that we're sure of the potency of the yeast.

The other part of the mystery centers around kneading. Perhaps if the word *stretching* were used instead, it would be less formidable a process. Once the dough is formed it needs to be made elastic by pulling, and while the classic technique is to pull a small amount toward you and then reverse the process, any variation that stretches the dough is effective. If you use an electric mixer and beat for four minutes at low speed, it is not necessary to knead for ten to twelve minutes as some recipes ask. A spirited seven minutes (with your favorite radio music for accompaniment) is sufficient.

However, if you begin to make bread regularly and to depend on its superior quality, you may find, as we did, a better way. While there are bread hooks that can be bought with good quality electric mixers, the bowls themselves hold flour for no more than three loaves of bread. As to the claims of the expensive food processors for bread making, this is plain silly, since their capacity allows for making only one loaf of bread.

But there is an inexpensive piece of equipment sold in hardware stores, a simple metal bucket with a hand-turned mixer. This makes kneading unnecessary, requires only four or five minutes of turning that anyone walking through the kitchen can be drafted to perform, and easily accommodates dough for six breads or more. Then, all you need is a freezer for storage, where bread keeps very well. Don't run out and buy a bread bucket now unless you've had some bread-making experience. After all, you may decide you don't have a spare minute in your life, much less a little time for bread. You should know, however, that it gets considerably easier each time you bake, whether by hand or with a mixer.

Once you've gotten your hands into bread making you'll

feel free to improvise, to add and subtract according to your individual taste. Note: It is impossible to give the exact amounts of flour in proportion to liquids. A little more or less will not appreciably affect the bread, but too little flour leaves the baker trying to detach the dough from his or her fingers rather than shaping it into handsome loaves. Much too much flour, on the other hand, makes for a heavy and proportionately less nutritious loaf.

The breads that follow are our basic breads, nutritious and good enough to really qualify as the Staff of Life.

• *Whole Wheat Bread* •
Makes 3 loaves

Have everything at least at room temperature, and don't be put off by what seems like a large number of ingredients.

⅔	cup warm, not hot, water
1	teaspoon sugar
2	packages dry yeast
3½	cups whole wheat flour
½	cup cracked wheat kernels (bulgur #1)
¼	cup wheat germ
⅓	cup soy flour (optional)
⅔	cup dry skim milk
3	teaspoons salt
2	cups lukewarm water
⅓	cup sunflower or corn oil
⅓	cup molasses
3	cups white unbleached flour

1. Place warm water and sugar in a glass 12 ounces or larger. Add yeast when the temperature is about 115°. Set aside in a warm place to rise and get foamy while you assemble the other ingredients, or for at least 5 minutes.

2. In the large bowl of an electric mixer stir together the whole wheat flour, wheat kernels, wheat germ, soy flour if you're using it, dry milk, salt, and water.

3. Using the same measuring cup for both, add the oil and

molasses in that order, so the molasses won't stick to the cup.

4. Add the yeast-water-sugar mix to the large bowl and beat at the lowest speed for about 4 minutes, slowly adding a cup of white flour. At the end of that time add the remainder of the white flour until the mix begins to climb up the beaters.

5. Stop the mixer and incorporate the remaining flour with a spoon. If the dough is still sticky, add small amounts of part white and whole wheat flour. Stop adding when the dough is manageable; that is, when it can be worked without sticking to your fingers.

6. Turn out the ball of dough onto a floured surface — wooden or Formica — and knead steadily for about 6 minutes, using a light sprinkling of flour on your hands, and occasionally adding more flour if some is needed.

7. Grease a large bowl and place the ball of dough in it, turning so that all sides are a bit oily. Cover the bowl with a damp clean cloth or an oiled piece of wax paper and then a towel. Place the bowl in a warmish (80° to 85°) spot. An oven with a pilot light is perfect.

8. Let the dough rise for about an hour or until it is almost doubled. Punch it down with your fist, and replace the bowl in the warming place. Let it rise again until doubled, about 50 minutes this time. (This last step, the second rising, is sometimes omitted, but it improves the bread's texture considerably.)

9. After the second rising, dump the dough onto the floured surface, knead it for a minute or so, and divide it in three parts. Roll out each piece about 9 inches in length, and then roll it up from the long end, jelly-roll fashion. Place each, seam side down, in a loaf pan greased with margarine, not oil. Return to the warming place for about 50 minutes or until the loaves are about double in height.

10. Bake in a pre-heated 350° oven for about an hour. Remove immediately from the pans by running a knife around the edge. Place the loaves on a wire rack to cool. Don't attempt to cut yeast bread when it is hot.

Of course bread can be made without an electric mixer. In

that case, it would be advisable to spend only a minute or two beating in the ingredients and to knead the dough for 8 to 10 minutes, instead of 6.

• *Oatmeal Bread* •

Use the same ingredients and procedure as Whole Wheat Bread, substituting 1½ cups of old-fashioned oatmeal for ¾ cup of white flour and ¾ cup of whole wheat.

• *White Bread* •
Makes 2 large loaves plus one small

⅔   cup warm water
1   teaspoon sugar
1   package plus 1 teaspoon yeast (refrigerate the re-
       mainder of the package)
¼   cup wheat germ
¼   cup soy flour (optional)
6–7 cups unbleached enriched flour
⅔   cup dry skim milk solids
3   teaspoons salt
4   tablespoons oil
3   tablespoons honey (add another tablespoon if soy flour
       is used)
2   cups lukewarm water, preferably water in which pota-
       toes have cooked; see variations following this recipe

1. Place warm water and sugar in a glass 12 ounces or larger. Add yeast when the water is about 115°. Set aside in a warm place to rise and get foamy while you assemble the other ingredients, or for at least 5 minutes.

2. In the large bowl of an electric mixer stir together 3 cups of the flour, the dry milk, wheat germ, soy flour if it is used, and salt.

3. Stir in the water, and, using the same measuring cup for both, add the oil and honey in that order, so the honey won't stick to the cup.

4. Add the yeast and water mixture and beat at the lowest

speed for about 3 minutes, slowly adding an additional cup of flour. Keep adding flour until the mix begins to climb up the beaters.

5. Stop the mixer and incorporate the remaining flour with a spoon. If the dough is still sticky, continue to add small amounts of flour until the dough can be worked without sticking to your fingers.

6. Turn out the ball of dough onto a floured surface — wooden or Formica — and knead steadily for about 7 minutes, using a light sprinkling of flour on your hands, and occasionally adding more flour if some is needed.

7. Grease a large bowl and place the dough in it, turning so that all sides are a bit oily. Cover the bowl with a damp, clean, thin cloth or an oiled piece of wax paper and then a towel. Place the bowl in a warmish (80° to 85°) spot. An oven with a pilot light is perfect.

8. Let the dough rise for about an hour or until it is almost doubled. Punch it down with your fist, cover, and replace the bowl in the warming place. Let it rise again until doubled, about 45 minutes.

9. After the second rising, dump the dough onto the floured surface, knead it for a minute or so, and divide it into two larger pieces and one small one. Flatten out the two larger pieces about 9 inches in length, and then roll them up from the long end, jelly-roll fashion. Place each, seam side down, in a margarine-greased loaf pan. Form the small piece into individual rolls or one round cottage loaf and place it in a greased pie tin. Return the pans to the warming place for about 50 minutes or until the loaves are about double in height.

10. Bake in a pre-heated 350° oven for about an hour. Remove immediately from the pans by running a knife around the edge. Place loaves on a wire rack to cool.

Variations: Our very favorite one is to substitute for part of the liquid one potato, peeled, cooked, and puréed with the water in which it was boiled. For white bread particularly the potato adds an excellent mellow flavor. You don't need to cook it especially. The day before breadmaking include some boiled potatoes in the menu, and simply cook one or two extra and save with the liquid. If the potato as well as the water is used, it should be put in the blender. Remember to let it come to at least room temperature before using.

Extras like sesame seeds for topping (or sliced onions) are among the many possibilities once the process becomes familiar. And remember the bread mixer. Six or seven loaves cooling on the counter, then waiting in the freezer, produce a wonderful feeling of nutritional self-sufficiency.

Appendixes

Nutritive Value of Foods

(Adapted from U.S. Department of Agriculture Bulletin #72)

[Dashes in the columns for nutrients show that no suitable value could be found although there is reason to believe that a measurable amount of the nutrient may be present]

Food, approximate measure, and weight (in grams)			Water	Food energy	Pro-tein	Fat
Milk, Cheese, Cream, Imitation Cream; Related Products						
		Grams	Per-cent	Calo-ries	Grams	Grams
Milk:						
Fluid:						
Whole, 3.5% fat	1 cup	244	87	160	9	9
Nonfat (skim)	1 cup	245	90	90	9	Trace
Partly skimmed, 2%	1 cup	246	87	145	10	5
Canned, concentrated, undiluted:						
Evaporated, unsweetened	1 cup	252	74	345	18	20
Condensed, sweetened	1 cup	306	27	980	25	27
Dry, nonfat instant	1 cup	104	4	375	37	1
Buttermilk:						
Fluid, cultured, made from skim milk	1 cup	245	90	90	8	Trace
Cheese:						
Natural:						
Blue or Roquefort type:						
Cubic inch	1 cu. in.	17	40	65	4	5
Cheddar:						
Cubic inch	1 cu. in.	17	37	70	4	6
Cottage, large or small curd:						
Creamed:						
Cup, curd pressed down	1 cup	245	78	260	33	10
Uncreamed:						
Cup, curd pressed down	1 cup	200	79	170	34	1
Cream:						
Cubic inch	1 cu. in.	16	51	60	1	6

[1] Value applies to unfortified product; the fortified product would be 2290 I.U.

| Fatty acids | | | | | | | | | | |
| | Unsaturated | | | | | | | | | |
Satu-rated (total)	Oleic	Lin-oleic	Carbo-hy-drate	Cal-cium	Iron	Vita-min A value	Thia-min	Ribo-flavin	Niacin	Ascor-bic acid
Grams	Grams	Grams	Grams	Milli-grams	Milli-grams	Inter-national units	Milli-grams	Milli-grams	Milli-grams	Milli-grams
5	3	Trace	12	288	0.1	350	0.07	0.41	0.2	2
—	—	—	12	296	.1	10	.09	.44	.2	2
3	2	Trace	15	352	.1	200	.10	.52	.2	2
11	7	1	24	635	.3	810	.10	.86	.5	3
15	9	1	166	802	.3	1,100	.24	1.16	.6	3
—	—	—	54	1,345	.6	[1]30	.36	1.85	.9	7
—	—	—	12	296	.1	10	.10	.44	.2	2
3	2	Trace	Trace	54	.1	210	.01	.11	.2	0
3	2	Trace	Trace	129	.2	230	.01	.08	Trace	0
6	3	Trace	7	230	.7	420	.07	.61	.2	0
Trace	Trace	Trace	5	180	.8	20	.06	.56	.2	0
3	2	Trace	Trace	10	Trace	250	Trace	.04	Trace	0

Food, approximate measure, and weight (in grams)		Grams	Water Per-cent	Food energy Calo-ries	Pro-tein Grams	Fat Grams
Parmesan, grated:						
Cup, pressed down	1 cup	140	17	655	60	43
Tablespoon	1 tbsp.	5	17	25	2	2
Swiss:						
Cubic inch	1 cu. in.	15	39	55	4	4
Pasteurized processed cheese:						
American:						
Cubic inch	1 cu. in.	18	40	65	4	5
Swiss:						
Cubic inch	1 cu. in.	18	40	65	5	5
Pasteurized process cheese food:						
American:						
Cubic inch	1 cu. in.	18	43	60	4	4
Cream:						
Half-and-half (cream and milk)	1 cup	242	80	325	8	28
Light, coffee or table	1 cup	240	72	505	7	49
Sour	1 cup	230	72	485	7	47
Whipped topping (pressurized)	1 cup	60	62	155	2	14
Whipping, unwhipped (volume about double when whipped):						
Heavy	1 cup	238	57	840	5	90
Imitation cream products (made with vegetable fat):						
Creamers:						
Powdered	1 cup	94	2	505	4	33
Liquid (frozen)	1 cup	245	77	345	3	27
Sour dressing (imitation sour cream) made with nonfat dry milk	1 cup	235	72	440	9	38
Whipped topping:						
Pressurized	1 cup	70	61	190	1	17
Milk beverages:						
Cocoa, homemade	1 cup	250	79	245	10	12
Chocolate-flavored drink made with skim milk and 2% added butterfat	1 cup	250	83	190	8	6

[2] Contributed largely from beta-corotene used for coloring.

Fatty acids			Carbo-hy-drate	Cal-cium	Iron	Vita-min A value	Thia-min	Ribo-flavin	Niacin	Ascor-bic acid
Satu-rated (total)	Unsaturated									
	Oleic	Lin-oleic								
Grams	Grams	Grams	Grams	Milli-grams	Milli-grams	Inter-national units	Milli-grams	Milli-grams	Milli-grams	Milli-grams
24	14	1	5	1,893	.7	1,760	.03	1.22	.3	0
1	Trace	Trace	Trace	68	Trace	60	Trace	.04	Trace	0
2	1	Trace	Trace	139	.1	170	Trace	.06	Trace	0
3	2	Trace	Trace	122	.2	210	Trace	.07	Trace	0
3	2	Trace	Trace	159	.2	200	Trace	.07	Trace	0
2	1	Trace	1	100	.1	170	Trace	.10	Trace	0
15	9	1	11	261	.1	1,160	.07	.39	.1	2
27	16	1	10	245	.1	2,020	.07	.36	.1	2
26	16	1	10	235	.1	1,930	.07	.35	.1	2
8	5	Trace	6	67	—	570	—	.04	—	—
50	30	3	7	179	.1	3,670	.05	.26	.1	2
31	1	0	52	21	.6	[2]200	—	—	Trace	—
25	1	0	25	29	—	[2]100	0	0	—	—
35	1	Trace	17	277	.1	10	.07	.38	.2	1
15	1	0	9	5	—	[2]340	—	0	—	—
7	4	Trace	27	295	1.0	400	.10	.45	.5	3
3	2	Trace	27	270	.5	210	.10	.40	.3	3

Food, approximate measure, and weight (in grams)		Grams	Water Per-cent	Food energy Calo-ries	Pro-tein Grams	Fat Grams
Milk desserts:						
Custard, baked	1 cup	265	77	305	14	15
Ice cream:						
Regular (approx. 10% fat)	1 cup	133	63	255	6	14
Rich (approx. 16% fat)	1 cup	148	63	330	4	24
Ice milk:						
Hardened	1 cup	131	67	200	6	7
Soft-serve	1 cup	175	67	265	8	9
Yoghurt:						
Made from partially skimmed milk	1 cup	245	89	125	8	4
Made from whole milk	1 cup	245	88	150	7	8
Eggs						
Eggs, large, 24 ounces per dozen:						
Whole, without shell	1 egg	50	74	80	6	6
White of egg	1 white	33	88	15	4	Trace
Yolk of egg	1 yolk	17	51	60	3	5
Scrambled with milk and fat	1 egg	64	72	110	7	8
Meat, Poultry, Fish, Shellfish; Related Products						
Bacon, broiled or fried, crisp	2 slices	15	8	90	5	8
Beef,[3] cooked:						
Cuts braised, simmered, or pot-roasted:						
Lean and fat	3 ounces	85	53	245	23	6
Hamburger (ground beef), broiled:						
Lean	3 ounces	85	60	185	23	10
Regular	3 ounces	85	54	245	21	17
Roast, oven-cooked, no liquid added:						
Relatively fat, such as rib:						
Lean and fat	3 ounces	85	40	375	17	34
Relatively lean, such as heel of round:						
Lean and fat	3 ounces	85	62	165	25	7

[3] Outer layer of fat on the cut was removed to within approximately ½-inch of the lean. Deposits of fat within the cut were not removed.

Fatty acids			Carbo-hy-drate	Cal-cium	Iron	Vita-min A value	Thia-min	Ribo-flavin	Niacin	Ascor-bic acid
Satu-rated (total)	Unsaturated									
	Oleic	Lin-oleic								
				Milli-grams	*Milli-grams*	*Inter-national units*	*Milli-grams*	*Milli-grams*	*Milli-grams*	*Milli-grams*
Grams	*Grams*	*Grams*	*Grams*							
7	5	1	29	297	1.1	930	.11	.50	.3	1
8	5	Trace	28	194	.1	590	.05	.28	.1	1
13	8	1	27	115	Trace	980	.03	.16	.1	1
4	2	Trace	29	204	.1	280	.07	.29	.1	1
5	3	Trace	39	273	.2	370	.09	.39	.2	2
2	1	Trace	13	294	.1	170	.10	.44	.2	2
5	3	Trace	12	272	.1	340	.07	.39	.2	2
2	3	Trace	Trace	27	1.1	590	.05	.15	Trace	0
—	—	—	Trace	3	Trace	0	Trace	.09	Trace	0
2	2	Trace	Trace	24	.9	580	.04	.07	Trace	0
3	3	Trace	1	51	1.1	690	.05	.18	Trace	0
3	4	1	1	2	.5	0	.08	.05	.8	—
8	7	Trace	0	10	2.9	30	.04	.18	3.5	—
5	4	Trace	0	10	3.0	20	.08	.20	5.1	—
8	8	Trace	0	9	2.7	30	.07	.18	4.6	—
16	15	1	0	8	2.2	70	.05	.13	3.1	—
3	3	Trace	0	11	3.2	10	.06	.19	4.5	—

Food, approximate measure, and weight (in grams)		Water	Food energy	Pro- tein	Fat
	Grams	Per- cent	Calo- ries	Grams	Grams
Steak, broiled:					
Relatively, fat, such as sirloin:					
Lean and fat	3 ounces	85	44	330	20	27
Beef and vegetable stew	1 cup	235	82	210	15	10
Beef potpie, baked, 4¼-inch diam., weight about 8 ounces	1 pie	227	55	560	23	33
Chicken, cooked:					
Flesh only, broiled	3 ounces	85	71	115	20	3
Breast, fried, ½ breast:					
Flesh and skin only	2.7 ounces	76	58	155	25	5
Drumstick, fried:					
Flesh and skin only	1.3 ounces	38	55	90	12	4
Chicken potpie, baked 4¼-inch diam., weight about 8 ounces	1 pie	227	57	535	23	31
Chili con carne, canned:					
With beans	1 cup	250	72	335	19	15
Lamb,[3] cooked:					
Chop, thick, with bone, broiled	1 chop, 4.8 ounces	137	47	400	25	33
Leg, roasted:					
Lean and fat	3 ounces	85	54	235	22	16
Shoulder, roasted:					
Lean and fat	3 ounces	85	50	285	18	23
Liver, beef, fried	2 ounces	57	57	130	15	6
Pork, cured, cooked:					
Ham, light cure, lean and fat, roasted	3 ounces	85	54	245	18	19
Luncheon meat:					
Boiled ham, sliced	2 ounces	57	59	135	11	10
Pork, fresh,[3] cooked:					
Chop, thick, with bone	1 chop, 3.5 ounces	98	42	260	16	21
Roast, oven-cooked, no liquid added:					
Lean and fat	3 ounces	85	46	310	21	24

[3] Outer layer of fat on the cut was removed to within approximately ½-inch of the lean. Deposits of fat within the cut were not removed.

Fatty acids										
Saturated (total)	Unsaturated		Carbohydrate	Calcium	Iron	Vitamin A value	Thiamin	Riboflavin	Niacin	Ascorbic acid
	Oleic	Linoleic								
Grams	*Grams*	*Grams*	*Grams*	*Milligrams*	*Milligrams*	*International units*	*Milligrams*	*Milligrams*	*Milligrams*	*Milligrams*
13	12	1	0	9	2.5	50	.05	.16	4.0	—
5	4	Trace	15	28	2.8	2,310	.13	.17	4.4	15
9	20	2	43	32	4.1	1,860	0.25	0.27	4.5	7
1	1	1	0	8	1.4	80	.05	.16	7.4	—
1	2	1	1	9	1.3	70	.04	.17	11.2	—
1	2	1	Trace	6	.9	50	.03	.15	2.7	—
10	15	3	42	68	3.0	3,020	.25	.26	4.1	5
7	7	Trace	30	80	4.2	150	.08	.18	3.2	—
18	12	1	0	10	1.5	—	.14	.25	5.6	—
9	6	Trace	0	9	1.4	—	.13	.23	4.7	—
13	8	1	0	9	1.0	—	.11	.20	4.0	—
—	—	—	3	6	5.0	30,280	.15	2.37	9.4	15
7	8	2	0	8	2.2	0	.40	.16	3.1	—
4	4	1	0	6	1.6	0	.25	.09	1.5	—
8	9	2	0	8	2.2	0	.63	.18	3.8	—
9	10	2	0	9	2.7	0	.78	.22	4.7	—

Food, approximate measure, and weight (in grams)		Water	Food energy	Pro-tein	Fat
		Grams	Per-cent	Calo-ries	Grams	Grams
Sausage:						
Bologna	2 slices	26	56	80	3	7
Braunschweiger	2 slices	20	53	65	3	5
Frankfurter	1 frank	56	57	170	7	15
Pork links	2 links	26	35	125	5	11
Salami, dry type	1 oz.	28	30	130	7	11
Veal, medium fat, cooked, bone removed:						
Cutlet	3 oz.	85	60	185	23	9
Roast	3 oz.	85	55	230	23	14
Fish and shellfish:						
Bluefish, baked with table fat	3 oz.	85	68	135	22	4
Clams:						
Raw, meat only	3 oz.	85	82	65	11	1
Crabmeat, canned	3 oz.	85	77	85	15	2
Fish sticks, breaded, cooked, frozen	10 sticks or 8 oz. pkg.	227	66	400	38	20
Haddock, breaded, fried	3 oz.	85	66	140	17	5
Oysters, raw	1 cup	240	85	160	20	4
Salmon, pink, canned	3 oz.	85	71	120	17	5
Sardines, Atlantic, canned in oil, drained solids	3 oz.	85	62	175	20	9
Shrimp, canned, meat	3 oz.	85	70	100	21	1
Swordfish, broiled with butter or margarine	3 oz.	85	65	150	24	5
Tuna, canned in oil, drained solids	3 oz.	85	61	170	24	7
Mature Dry Beans and Peas, Nuts, Peanuts; Related Products						
Almonds, shelled, whole kernels	1 cup	142	5	850	26	77
Beans, dry:						
Cooked, drained:						
Great Northern	1 cup	180	69	210	14	1
Navy (pea)	1 cup	190	69	225	15	1

[4]If bones are discarded, value will be greatly reduced.

Fatty acids			Carbo-hy-drate	Cal-cium	Iron	Vita-min A value	Thia-min	Ribo-flavin	Niacin	Ascor-bic acid
Satu-rated (total)	Unsaturated									
	Oleic	Lin-oleic								
Grams	Grams	Grams	Grams	Milli-grams	Milli-grams	Inter-national units	Milli-grams	Milli-grams	Milli-grams	Milli-grams
—	—	—	Trace	2	.5	—	.04	.06	.7	—
—	—	—	Trace	2	1.2	1,310	.03	.29	1.6	—
—	—	—	1	3	.8	—	.08	.11	1.4	—
4	5	1	Trace	2	.6	0	.21	.09	1.0	—
—	—	—	Trace	4	1.0	—	.10	.07	1.5	—
5	4	Trace	—	9	2.7	—	.06	.21	4.6	—
7	6	Trace	0	10	2.9	—	.11	.26	6.6	—
—	—	—	0	25	.6	40	.09	.08	1.6	—
—	—	—	2	59	5.2	90	.08	.15	1.1	8
—	—	—	1	38	.7	—	.07	.07	1.6	—
5	4	10	15	25	0.9	—	0.09	0.16	3.6	—
1	3	Trace	5	34	1.0	—	.03	.06	2.7	2
—	—	—	8	226	13.2	740	.33	.43	6.0	—
1	1	Trace	0	[4]167	.7	60	.03	.16	6.8	—
—	—	—	0	372	2.5	190	.02	.17	4.6	—
—	—	—	1	98	2.6	50	.01	.03	1.5	—
—	—	—	0	23	1.1	1,750	.03	.04	9.3	—
2	1	1	0	7	1.6	70	.04	.10	10.1	—
6	52	15	28	332	6.7	0	.34	1.31	5.0	Trace
—	—	—	38	90	4.9	0	.25	.13	1.3	0
—	—	—	40	95	5.1	0	.27	.13	1.3	0

Food, approximate measure, and weight (in grams)		Water	Food energy	Pro-tein	Fat
	Grams	Per-cent	Calo-ries	Grams	Grams
Canned, solids and liquid:					
Pork and tomato sauce	1 cup	255	71	310	16	7
Red kidney	1 cup	255	76	230	15	1
Cashew nuts, roasted	1 cup	140	5	785	24	64
Coconut, fresh, meat only:					
Shredded or grated, firmly packed	1 cup	130	51	450	5	46
Cowpeas or blackeye peas, dry, cooked	1 cup	248	80	190	13	1
Peanuts, roasted, salted, halves	1 cup	144	2	840	37	72
Peanut butter	1 tbsp.	16	2	95	4	8
Peas, split, dry, cooked	1 cup	250	70	290	20	1
Pecans, halves	1 cup	108	3	740	10	77
Walnuts, chopped	1 cup	126	3	790	26	75

Vegetables and Vegetable Products

Asparagus, green:					
Cooked, drained	4 spears	60	94	10	1	Trace
Canned, solids and liquid	1 cup	244	94	45	5	1
Beans:					
Lima, cooked, drained	1 cup	170	71	190	13	1
Snap Green:					
Cooked, drained	1 cup	125	92	30	2	Trace
Canned, solids and liquid	1 cup	239	94	45	2	Trace
Sprouted mung beans, cooked, drained	1 cup	125	91	35	4	Trace
Beets:					
Cooked, drained	2 beets	100	91	30	1	Trace
Beet greens, leaves and stems, cooked, drained	1 cup	145	94	25	3	Trace
Broccoli, cooked, drained:					
Whole stalks, medium size	1 stalk	180	91	45	6	1
Chopped, yield from 10-oz. frozen pkg.	1⅜ cups	250	92	65	7	1
Brussels sprouts, 7–8 per cup, cooked	1 cup	155	88	55	7	1

Fatty acids										
Saturated (total)	Unsaturated		Carbohydrate	Calcium	Iron	Vitamin A value	Thiamin	Riboflavin	Niacin	Ascorbic acid
	Oleic	Linoleic								
Grams	Grams	Grams	Grams	Milligrams	Milligrams	International units	Milligrams	Milligrams	Milligrams	Milligrams
2	3	1	49	138	4.6	330	.20	.08	1.5	5
—	—	—	42	74	4.6	10	.13	.10	1.5	—
11	45	4	41	53	5.3	140	.60	.35	2.5	—
39	3	Trace	12	17	2.2	0	.07	.03	.7	4
—	—	—	34	42	3.2	20	.41	.11	1.1	Trace
16	31	21	27	107	3.0	—	.46	.19	24.7	0
2	4	2	3	9	.3	—	.02	.02	2.4	0
—	—	—	52	28	4.2	100	.37	.22	2.2	—
5	48	15	16	79	2.6	140	.93	.14	1.0	2
4	26	36	19	Trace	7.6	380	.28	.14	.9	—
—	—	—	2	13	.4	540	.10	.11	.8	16
—	—	—	7	44	4.1	1,240	.15	.22	2.0	37
—	—	—	34	80	4.3	480	.31	.17	2.2	29
—	—	—	7	63	.8	680	.09	.11	.6	15
—	—	—	10	81	2.9	690	.07	.10	.7	10
—	—	—	7	21	1.1	30	.11	.13	.9	8
—	—	—	7	14	.5	20	.03	.04	.3	6
—	—	—	5	144	2.8	7,400	.10	.22	.4	22
—	—	—	8	158	1.4	4,500	.16	.36	1.4	162
—	—	—	12	135	1.8	6,500	.15	.30	1.3	143
—	—	—	10	50	1.7	810	.12	.22	1.2	135

Food, approximate measure, and weight (in grams)		Grams	Water Per-cent	Food energy Calo-ries	Pro-tein Grams	Fat Grams
Cabbage:						
Raw:						
Coarsely shredded	1 cup	70	92	15	1	Trace
Cooked	1 cup	145	94	30	2	Trace
Red, raw, coarsely shredded	1 cup	70	90	20	1	Trace
Carrots:						
Raw:						
Whole, 5½ by 1 inch	1 carrot	50	88	20	1	Trace
Cooked, diced	1 cup	145	91	45	1	Trace
Cauliflower, cooked, flowerbuds	1 cup	120	93	25	3	Trace
Celery, raw:						
Pieces, diced	1 cup	100	94	15	1	Trace
Collards, cooked	1 cup	190	91	55	5	1
Corn, sweet:						
Cooked [5]	1 ear	140	74	70	3	1
Canned, solids and liquid	1 cup	256	81	170	5	2
Cucumbers:						
Raw, pared	1 cucum-ber	207	96	30	1	Trace
Raw	6 slices	50	96	5	Trace	Trace
Endive, curly (including escarole)	2 ounces	57	93	10	1	Trace
Kale, leaves including stems, cooked	1 cup	110	91	30	4	1
Lettuce, raw:						
Butterhead, as Boston types; head, 4-inch diameter	1 head	220	95	30	3	Trace
Crisphead, as Iceberg; head, 4¾-inch diameter	1 head	454	96	60	4	Trace
Looseleaf, or bunching varieties, leaves	2 large	50	94	10	1	Trace
Mushrooms, canned, solids and liquid	1 cup	244	93	40	5	Trace
Mustard greens, cooked	1 cup	140	93	35	3	1
Okra, cooked, pod 3 by ⅝ inch	8 pods	85	91	25	2	Trace

[5] Measure and weight apply to entire vegetable or fruit including parts not usually eaten.

[6] Based on yellow varieties; white varieties contain only a trace of cryptoxanthin and carotenes, the pigments in corn that have biological activity.

Fatty acids			Carbo-hy-drate	Cal-cium	Iron	Vita-min A value	Thia-min	Ribo-flavin	Niacin	Ascor-bic acid
Satu-rated (total)	Unsaturated									
	Oleic	Lin-oleic								
Grams	Grams	Grams	Grams	Milli-grams	Milli-grams	Inter-national units	Milli-grams	Milli-grams	Milli-grams	Milli-grams
—	—	—	4	34	.3	90	.04	.04	.2	33
—	—	—	6	64	.4	190	.06	.06	.4	48
—	—	—	5	29	.6	30	.06	.04	.3	43
—	—	—	5	18	.4	5,500	.03	.03	.3	4
—	—	—	10	48	.9	15,220	.08	.07	.7	9
—	—	—	5	25	.8	70	.11	.10	.7	66
—	—	—	4	39	.3	240	.03	.03	.3	9
—	—	—	9	289	1.1	10,260	.27	.37	2.4	87
—	—	—	16	2	.5	[6]310	.09	.08	1.0	7
—	—	—	40	10	1.0	[6]690	.07	.12	2.3	13
—	—	—	7	35	.6	Trace	.07	.09	.4	23
—	—	—	2	8	.2	Trace	.02	.02	.1	6
—	—	—	2	46	1.0	1,870	0.04	0.08	0.3	6
—	—	—	4	147	1.3	8,140	—	—	—	68
—	—	—	6	77	4.4	2,130	.14	.13	.6	18
—	—	—	13	91	2.3	1,500	.29	.27	1.3	29
—	—	—	2	34	.7	950	.03	.04	.2	9
—	—	—	6	15	1.2	Trace	.04	.60	4.8	4
—	—	—	6	193	2.5	8,120	.11	.19	.9	68
—	—	—	5	78	.4	420	.11	.15	.8	17

Food, approximate measure, and weight (in grams)		Water	Food energy	Protein	Fat
		Grams	*Percent*	*Calories*	*Grams*	*Grams*
Onions:						
Mature:						
Raw, onion 2½-inch diameter	1 onion	110	89	40	2	Trace
Cooked	1 cup	210	92	60	3	Trace
Young green, small, without tops	6 onions	50	88	20	1	Trace
Parsley, raw, chopped	1 tablespoon	4	85	Trace	Trace	Trace
Parsnips, cooked	1 cup	155	82	100	2	1
Peas, green:						
Cooked	1 cup	160	82	115	9	1
Canned, solids and liquid	1 cup	249	83	165	9	1
Peppers, sweet:						
Raw, about 5 per pound	1 pod	74	93	15	1	Trace
Cooked, boiled, drained	1 pod	73	95	15	1	Trace
Potatoes, medium (about 3 per pound raw):						
Baked	1 potato	99	75	90	3	Trace
Boiled:						
Peeled after boiling	1 potato	136	80	105	3	Trace
French-fried, piece 2 by ½ by ½ inch:						
Cooked in deep fat	10 pieces	57	45	155	2	7
Frozen, heated	10 pieces	57	53	125	2	5
Mashed:						
Milk added	1 cup	195	83	125	4	1
Milk and butter added	1 cup	195	80	185	4	8
Potato chips, medium, 2-inch diameter	10 chips	20	2	115	1	8
Pumpkin, canned	1 cup	228	90	75	2	1
Radishes, raw, small, without tops	4 radishes	40	94	5	Trace	Trace
Spinach:						
Cooked	1 cup	180	92	40	5	1
Squash:						
Cooked:						
Summer, diced	1 cup	210	96	30	2	Trace
Winter, baked	1 cup	205	81	130	4	1

Fatty acids										
Saturated (total)	Unsaturated		Carbohydrate	Calcium	Iron	Vitamin A value	Thiamin	Riboflavin	Niacin	Ascorbic acid
	Oleic	Linoleic								
Grams	*Grams*	*Grams*	*Grams*	*Milligrams*	*Milligrams*	*International units*	*Milligrams*	*Milligrams*	*Milligrams*	*Milligrams*
—	—	—	10	30	.6	40	.04	.04	.2	11
—	—	—	14	50	.8	80	.06	.06	.4	14
—	—	—	5	20	.3	Trace	.02	.02	.2	12
—	—	—	Trace	8	.2	340	Trace	.01	Trace	7
—	—	—	23	70	.9	50	.11	.12	.2	16
—	—	—	19	37	2.9	860	.44	.17	3.7	33
—	—	—	31	50	4.2	1,120	.23	.13	2.2	22
—	—	—	4	7	.5	310	.06	.06	.4	94
—	—	—	3	7	.4	310	.05	.05	.4	70
—	—	—	21	9	.7	Trace	.10	.04	1.7	20
—	—	—	23	10	.8	Trace	.13	.05	2.0	22
2	2	4	20	9	.7	Trace	.07	.04	1.8	12
1	1	2	19	5	1.0	Trace	.08	.01	1.5	12
—	—	—	25	47	.8	50	.16	.10	2.0	19
4	3	Trace	24	47	.8	330	.16	.10	1.9	18
2	2	4	10	8	.4	Trace	.04	.01	1.0	3
—	—	—	18	57	.9	14,590	.07	.12	1.3	12
—	—	—	1	12	.4	Trace	.01	.01	.1	10
—	—	—	6	167	4.0	14,580	.13	.25	1.0	50
—	—	—	7	52	.8	820	.10	.16	1.6	21
—	—	—	32	57	1.6	8,610	.10	.27	1.4	27

Food, approximate measure, and weight (in grams)		Water	Food energy	Pro-tein	Fat
		Grams	*Per-cent*	*Calo-ries*	*Grams* *Grams*

		Grams	*Per-cent*	*Calo-ries*	*Grams*	*Grams*
Sweet potatoes:						
Cooked, medium, 5 by 2 inches, weight raw about 6 ounces:						
Baked	1 sweet potato	110	64	155	2	1
Candied, 3½ by 2¼ inches	1 sweet potato	175	60	295	2	6
Canned, vacuum or solid pack	1 cup	218	72	235	4	Trace
Tomatoes:						
Raw, approx. 3-in. diam. 2⅛ in. high	1 tomato	200	94	40	2	Trace
Canned, solids and liquid	1 cup	241	94	50	2	1
Tomato catsup:						
Tablespoon	1 tbsp.	15	69	15	Trace	Trace
Tomato juice, canned:						
Glass (6 fl. oz.)	1 glass	182	94	35	2	Trace
Turnips, cooked, diced	1 cup	155	94	35	1	Trace
Fruits and Fruit Products						
Apples, raw (about 3 per lb.)[5]	1 apple	150	85	70	Trace	Trace
Apple juice, bottled or canned	1 cup	248	88	120	Trace	Trace
Applesauce, canned:						
Sweetened	1 cup	255	76	230	1	Trace
Unsweetened or artificially sweetened	1 cup	244	88	100	1	Trace
Apricots:						
Raw (about 12 per lb.)[5]	3 apricots	114	85	55	1	Trace
Canned in heavy sirup	1 cup	259	77	220	2	Trace
Dried, uncooked (40 halves per cup)	1 cup	150	25	390	8	1
Cooked, unsweetened, fruit and liquid	1 cup	285	76	240	5	1
Apricot nectar, canned	1 cup	251	85	140	1	Trace

[5] Measure and weight apply to entire vegetable or fruit including parts not usually eaten.
[7] Year-round average. Samples marketed from November through May, average 20 milligrams per 200-gram tomato; from June through October, around 52 milligrams.

Fatty acids										
Unsaturated										
Saturated (total)	Oleic	Linoleic	Carbohydrate	Calcium	Iron	Vitamin A value	Thiamin	Riboflavin	Niacin	Ascorbic acid
Grams	Grams	Grams	Grams	Milligrams	Milligrams	International units	Milligrams	Milligrams	Milligrams	Milligrams
—	—	—	36	44	1.0	8,910	.10	.07	.7	24
2	3	1	60	65	1.6	11,030	0.10	0.08	0.8	17
—	—	—	54	54	1.7	17,000	.10	.10	1.4	30
—	—	—	9	24	.9	1,640	.11	.07	1.3	[7]42
—	—	—	10	14	1.2	2,170	.12	.07	1.7	41
—	—	—	4	3	.1	210	.01	.01	.2	2
—	—	—	8	13	1.6	1,460	.09	.05	1.5	29
—	—	—	8	54	.6	Trace	.06	.08	.5	34
—	—	—	18	8	.4	50	.04	.02	.1	3
—	—	—	30	15	1.5	—	.02	.05	.2	2
—	—	—	61	10	1.3	100	.05	.03	.1	[8]3
—	—	—	26	10	1.2	100	.05	.02	.1	[8]2
—	—	—	14	18	.5	2,890	.03	.04	.7	10
—	—	—	57	28	.8	4,510	.05	.06	.9	10
—	—	—	100	100	8.2	16,350	.02	.23	4.9	19
—	—	—	62	63	5.1	8,550	.01	.13	2.8	8
—	—	—	37	23	.5	2,380	.03	.03	.5	[8]8

[8]This is the amount from the fruit. Additional ascorbic acid may be added by the manufacturer. Refer to the label for this information.

Food, approximate measure, and weight (in grams)		Grams	Water Per-cent	Food energy Calo-ries	Pro-tein Grams	Fat Grams
Avocados, whole fruit, raw:[5]						
California (mid- and late-winter; diam. 3⅛ in.)	1 avocado	284	74	370	5	37
Florida (late summer, fall; diam. 3⅝ in.)	1 avocado	454	78	390	4	33
Bananas, raw, medium size[5]	1 banana	175	76	100	1	Trace
Blueberries, raw	1 cup	140	83	85	1	1
Cantaloupes, raw; medium, 5-inch diameter	½ melon	385	91	60	1	Trace
Cherries, canned, red, sour, pitted, water pack	1 cup	244	88	105	2	Trace
Cranberry juice cocktail, canned	1 cup	250	83	165	Trace	Trace
Cranberry sauce, sweetened, canned, strained	1 cup	277	62	405	Trace	1
Dates, pitted, cut	1 cup	178	22	490	4	1
Figs, dried, large, 2 by 1 in.	1 fig	21	23	60	1	Trace
Fruit cocktail, canned, in heavy sirup	1 cup	256	80	195	1	Trace
Grapefruit:						
Raw, medium, 3¾-in. diam.[5]						
White	½ grape-fruit	241	89	45	1	Trace
Pink or red	½ grape-fruit	241	89	50	1	Trace
Canned, sirup pack	1 cup	254	81	180	2	Trace
Grapefruit juice:						
Fresh	1 cup	246	90	95	1	Trace
Canned, white:						
Unsweetened	1 cup	247	89	100	1	Trace
Sweetened	1 cup	250	86	130	1	Trace
Frozen, concentrate, unsweetened:						
Diluted	1 cup	247	89	100	1	Trace
Grapes, raw:[5]						
American type (slip skin)	1 cup	153	82	65	1	1

[5] Measure and weight apply to entire vegetable or fruit including parts not usually eaten.

[9] Value for varieties with orange-colored flesh; value for varieties with green flesh would be about 540 I.U.

	Fatty acids									
	Unsaturated									
Satu-rated (total)	Oleic	Lin-oleic	Carbo-hy-drate	Cal-cium	Iron	Vita-min A value	Thia-min	Ribo-flavin	Niacin	Ascor-bic acid
Grams	Grams	Grams	Grams	Milli-grams	Milli-grams	Inter-national units	Milli-grams	Milli-grams	Milli-grams	Milli-grams
7	17	5	13	22	1.3	630	.24	.43	3.5	30
7	15	4	27	30	1.8	880	.33	.61	4.9	43
—	—	—	26	10	.8	230	.06	.07	.8	12
—	—	—	21	21	1.4	140	.04	.08	.6	20
—	—	—	14	27	.8	[9] 6,540	.08	.06	1.2	63
—	—	—	26	37	.7	1,660	.07	.05	.5	12
—	—	—	42	13	.8	Trace	.03	.03	.1	[10] 40
—	—	—	104	17	.6	60	.03	.03	.1	6
—	—	—	130	105	5.3	90	.16	.17	3.9	0
—	—	—	15	26	.6	20	.02	.02	.1	0
—	—	—	50	23	1.0	360	.05	.03	1.3	5
—	—	—	12	19	0.5	10	0.05	0.02	0.2	44
—	—	—	13	20	0.5	540	0.05	0.02	0.2	44
—	—	—	45	33	.8	30	.08	.05	.5	76
—	—	—	23	22	.5	([11])	.09	.04	.4	92
—	—	—	24	20	1.0	20	.07	.04	.4	84
—	—	—	32	20	1.0	20	.07	.04	.4	78
—	—	—	24	25	.2	20	.10	.04	.5	96
—	—	—	15	15	.4	100	.05	.03	.2	3

[10] Value listed is based on products with label stating 30 milligrams per 6 fl. oz. serving.
[11] For white-fleshed varieties value is about 20 I.U. per cup; for red-fleshed varieties, 1,080 I.U. per cup.

Food, approximate measure, and weight (in grams)		Water	Food energy	Pro-tein	Fat
		Per-	*Calo-*		
	Grams	*cent*	*ries*	*Grams*	*Grams*
European type (adherent skin)	1 cup	160	81	95	1	Trace
Grape juice:					
Canned or bottled	1 cup	253	83	165	1	Trace
Lemons, raw, 2⅛-inch. diam.	1 lemon	110	90	20	1	Trace
Lemonade concentrate:					
Diluted	1 cup	248	88	110	Trace	Trace
Lime juice:					
Fresh	1 cup	246	90	65	1	Trace
Limeade concentrate, frozen:					
Diluted	1 cup	247	90	100	Trace	Trace
Oranges, raw, 2⅝-in. diam.	1 orange	180	86	65	1	Trace
Orange juice, fresh	1 cup	248	88	110	2	1
Canned, unsweetened	1 cup	249	87	120	2	Trace
Frozen concentrate:					
Diluted	1 cup	249	87	120	2	Trace
Peaches:					
Raw:					
Whole, medium, 2-inch diameter	1 peach	114	89	35	1	Trace
Canned, yellow-fleshed, solids and liquid:					
Sirup pack, heavy:					
Halves or slices	1 cup	257	79	200	1	Trace
Water pack	1 cup	245	91	75	1	Trace
Pears:					
Raw, 3 by 2½-inch diameter[5]	1 pear	182	83	100	1	1
Canned, solids and liquid:					
Sirup pack, heavy:					
Halves or slices	1 cup	255	80	195	1	1
Pineapple:					
Raw, diced	1 cup	140	85	75	1	Trace
Canned, heavy sirup pack, solids and liquid:					
Crushed	1 cup	260	80	195	1	Trace
Sliced, slices and juice	2 small or 1 large	122	80	90	Trace	Trace
Pineapple juice, canned	1 cup	249	86	135	1	Trace

[5] Measure and weight apply to entire vegetable or fruit including parts not usually eaten.

[8] This is the amount from the fruit. Additional ascorbic acid may be added by the manufacturer. Refer to the label for this information.

Fatty acids										
Satu-rated (total)	Unsaturated		Carbo-hy-drate	Cal-cium	Iron	Vita-min A value	Thia-min	Ribo-flavin	Niacin	Ascor-bic acid
	Oleic	Lin-oleic								
Grams	Grams	Grams	Grams	Milli-grams	Milli-grams	Inter-national units	Milli-grams	Milli-grams	Milli-grams	Milli-grams
—	—	—	25	17	.6	140	.07	.04	.4	6
—	—	—	42	28	.8	—	.10	.05	.5	Trace
—	—	—	6	19	.4	10	.03	.01	.1	39
—	—	—	28	2	Trace	Trace	Trace	.02	.2	17
—	—	—	22	22	.5	20	.05	.02	.2	79
—	—	—	27	2	Trace	Trace	Trace	Trace	Trace	5
—	—	—	16	54	.5	260	.13	.05	.5	66
—	—	—	26	27	.5	500	.22	.07	1.0	124
—	—	—	28	25	1.0	500	.17	.05	.7	100
—	—	—	29	25	.2	550	.22	.02	1.0	120
—	—	—	10	9	.5	[13]1,320	.02	.05	1.0	7
—	—	—	52	10	.8	1,100	.02	.06	1.4	7
—	—	—	20	10	.7	1,100	.02	.06	1.4	7
—	—	—	25	13	.5	30	.04	.07	.2	7
—	—	—	50	13	.5	Trace	.03	.05	.3	4
—	—	—	19	24	.7	100	.12	.04	.3	24
—	—	—	50	29	.8	120	.20	.06	.5	17
—	—	—	24	13	.4	50	.09	.03	.2	8
—	—	—	34	37	.7	120	.12	.04	.5	[8]22

[13] Based on yellow-fleshed varieties; for white-fleshed varieties value is about 50 I.U. per 114-gram peach and 80 I.U. per cup of sliced peaches.

Food, approximate measure, and weight (in grams)			Water	Food energy	Pro-tein	Fat
		Grams	Per-cent	Calo-ries	Grams	Grams
Plums, all except prunes:						
Raw, 2-inch diameter	1 plum	60	87	25	Trace	Trace
Canned, sirup pack (Italian prunes):						
Plums (with pits) and juice[5]	1 cup	256	77	205	1	Trace
Prunes, dried, "softenized," medium:						
Uncooked[5]	4 prunes	32	28	70	1	Trace
Cooked, unsweetened	1 cup	270	66	295	2	1
Prune juice, canned or bottled	1 cup	256	80	200	1	Trace
Raisins, seedless:						
Packaged, ½ oz.	1 pkg.	14	18	40	Trace	Trace
Cup, pressed down	1 cup	165	18	480	4	Trace
Raspberries, red:						
Raw	1 cup	123	84	70	1	1
Frozen, 10-ounce carton, not thawed	1 carton	284	74	275	2	1
Strawberries:						
Raw, capped	1 cup	149	90	55	1	1
Frozen, 10-ounce carton	1 carton	284	71	310	1	1
Tangerines, raw, medium, 2⅜-in. diam.	1 tanger-ine	116	87	40	1	Trace
Watermelon, raw, wedge, 4 by 8 inches	1 wedge	925	93	115	2	1
Grain Products						
Bagel, 3-in. diam.:	1 bagel	55	32	165	6	2
Barley, pearled, light, uncooked	1 cup	200	11	700	16	2
Biscuits, baking powder from home recipe with enriched flour, 2-in. diam.	1 biscuit	28	27	105	2	5
Biscuits, baking powder from mix, 2-in. diam.	1 biscuit	28	28	90	2	3
Bran flakes (40% bran), added thiamin and iron	1 cup	35	3	105	4	1
Breads:						
Boston brown bread, slice 3 by ¾ in.	1 slice	48	45	100	3	1

[5] Measure and weight apply to entire vegetable or fruit including parts not usually eaten.

Fatty acids										
Saturated (total)	Unsaturated		Carbo-hy-drate	Cal-cium	Iron	Vita-min A value	Thia-min	Ribo-flavin	Niacin	Ascor-bic acid
	Oleic	Lin-oleic								
Grams	Grams	Grams	Grams	Milli-grams	Milli-grams	Inter-national units	Milli-grams	Milli-grams	Milli-grams	Milli-grams
—	—	—	7	7	.3	140	.02	.02	.3	3
—	—	—	53	22	2.2	2,970	.05	.05	.9	4
—	—	—	18	14	1.1	440	.02	.04	.4	1
—	—	—	78	60	4.5	1,860	.08	.18	1.7	2
—	—	—	49	36	10.5	—	.03	.03	1.0	[8]5
—	—	—	11	9	.5	Trace	.02	.01	.1	Trace
—	—	—	128	102	5.8	30	.18	.13	.8	2
—	—	—	17	27	1.1	160	.04	.11	1.1	31
—	—	—	70	37	1.7	200	.06	.17	1.7	59
—	—	—	13	31	1.5	90	.04	.10	1.0	88
—	—	—	79	40	2.0	90	.06	.17	1.5	150
—	—	—	10	34	.3	360	.05	.02	.1	27
—	—	—	27	30	2.1	2,510	13	.13	.7	30
—	—	—	28	9	1.2	30	0.14	0.10	1.2	0
Trace	1	1	158	32	4.0	0	.24	.10	6.2	0
1	2	1	13	34	.4	Trace	.06	.06	.1	Trace
1	1	1	15	19	.6	Trace	.08	.07	.6	Trace
—	—	—	28	25	12.3	0	.14	.06	2.2	0
—	—	—	22	43	.9	0	.05	.03	.6	0

[8] This is the amount from the fruit. Additional ascorbic acid may be added by the manufacturer. Refer to the label for this information.

Food, approximate measure, and weight (in grams)		Grams	Water Per-cent	Food energy Calo-ries	Pro-tein Grams	Fat Grams
Cracked-wheat bread	1 slice	25	35	65	2	1
Raisin bread	1 slice	25	35	65	2	1
Rye bread:						
American, light	1 slice	25	36	60	2	Trace
White bread, enriched:[15]						
Soft-crumb type	1 slice	25	36	70	2	1
Firm-crumb type	1 slice	23	35	65	2	1
Whole-wheat bread, soft-crumb type	1 slice	28	36	65	3	1
Whole-wheat bread, firm-crumb type	1 slice	25	36	60	3	1
Cakes made from cake mixes:						
Angelfood:						
Piece, 1/12 of 10-in. diam. cake	1 piece	53	34	135	3	Trace
Devil's food, 2-layer, with chocolate icing:						
Piece, 1/16 of 9-in. diam. cake	1 piece	69	24	235	3	9
Gingerbread:						
Piece, 1/9 of 8-in. square cake	1 piece	63	37	175	2	4
White, 2-layer, with chocolate icing:						
Piece, 1/16 of 9-in. diam. cake	1 piece	71	21	250	3	8
Cakes made from home recipes:[16]						
Boston cream pie; piece 1/12 of 8-in. diam.	1 piece	69	35	210	4	6
Fruitcake, dark, made with enriched flour:						
Slice, 1/30 of 8-in. loaf	1 slice	15	18	55	1	2
Pound:						
Slice, ½-in. thick	1 slice	30	17	140	2	9
Sponge:						
Piece, 1/12 of 10-in. diam. cake	1 piece	66	32	195	5	4
Yellow, 2-layer, without icing:						
Piece, 1/16 of 9-in. diam. cake	1 piece	54	24	200	2	7

[15] Values for iron, thiamin, riboflavin, and niacin per pound of unenriched white bread would be as follows:

	Iron Milligrams	Thiamin Milligrams	Riboflavin Milligrams	Niacin Milligrams
Soft crumb	3.2	.31	.39	5.0
Firm crumb	3.2	.32	.59	4.1

Fatty acids										
Saturated (total)	Unsaturated		Carbohydrate	Calcium	Iron	Vitamin A value	Thiamin	Riboflavin	Niacin	Ascorbic acid
	Oleic	Linoleic								
Grams	Grams	Grams	Grams	Milligrams	Milligrams	International units	Milligrams	Milligrams	Milligrams	Milligrams
—	—	—	13	22	.3	Trace	.03	.02	.3	Trace
—	—	—	13	18	.3	Trace	.01	.02	.2	Trace
—	—	—	13	19	.4	0	.05	.02	.4	0
—	—	—	13	21	.6	Trace	.06	.05	.6	Trace
—	—	—	12	22	.6	Trace	.06	.05	.6	Trace
—	—	—	14	24	.8	Trace	.09	.03	.8	Trace
—	—	—	12	25	.8	Trace	.06	.03	.7	Trace
—	—	—	32	50	.2	0	Trace	.06	.1	0
3	4	1	40	41	.6	100	.02	.06	.2	Trace
1	2	1	32	57	1.0	Trace	.02	.06	.5	Trace
3	3	1	45	70	.4	40	.01	.06	.1	Trace
2	3	1	34	46	.3	140	.02	.08	.1	Trace
Trace	1	Trace	9	11	.4	20	.02	.02	.1	Trace
2	4	1	14	6	.2	80	.01	.03	.1	0
1	2	Trace	36	20	.8	300	.03	.09	.1	Trace
2	3	1	32	39	.2	80	.01	.04	.1	Trace

[16] Unenriched cake flour used unless otherwise specified.

Food, approximate measure, and weight (in grams)			Water	Food energy	Pro-tein	Fat
		Grams	Per-cent	Calo-ries	Grams	Grams
Yellow, 2-layer, with chocolate icing:						
Piece, ¹/₁₆ of 9-in. diam. cake	1 piece	75	21	275	3	10
Cookies:						
Brownies with nuts:						
Made from home recipe with enriched flour	1 brownie	20	10	95	1	6
Made from mix	1 brownie	20	11	85	1	4
Chocolate chip:						
Made from home recipe with enriched flour	1 cookie	10	3	50	1	3
Commercial	1 cookie	10	3	50	1	2
Fig bars, commercial	1 cookie	14	14	50	1	1
Sandwich, chocolate or vanilla, commercial	1 cookie	10	2	50	1	2
Corn flakes, added nutrients:						
Plain	1 cup	25	4	100	2	Trace
Sugar-covered	1 cup	40	2	155	2	Trace
Corn muffins, made with enriched degermed cornmeal and enriched flour; muffin 2⅜-in. diam.	1 muffin	40	33	125	3	4
Corn muffins, made with mix, egg, and milk; muffin 2⅜-in. diam.	1 muffin	40	30	130	3	4
Crackers:						
Graham, 2½-in. square	4 crackers	28	6	110	2	3
Saltines	4 crackers	11	4	50	1	1
Doughnuts, cake type	1 dough-nut	32	24	125	1	6
Farina, quick-cooking, enriched, cooked	1 cup	245	89	105	3	Trace

[17] This value is based on product made from yellow varieties of corn; white varieties contain only a trace.

[18] Based on product made with enriched flour. With unenriched flour, approximate values per doughnut are: Iron, 0.2 milligram; thiamin, 0.01 milligram; riboflavin, 0.03 milligram; niacin, 0.2 milligram.

Saturated (total)	Fatty acids		Carbohydrate	Calcium	Iron	Vitamin A value	Thiamin	Riboflavin	Niacin	Ascorbic acid
	Unsaturated									
	Oleic	Linoleic								
Grams	Grams	Grams	Grams	Milligrams	Milligrams	International units	Milligrams	Milligrams	Milligrams	Milligrams
3	4	1	45	51	.5	120	.02	.06	.2	Trace
1	3	1	10	8	.4	40	.04	.02	.1	Trace
1	2	1	13	9	.4	20	.03	.02	.1	Trace
1	1	1	6	4	0.2	10	0.01	0.01	0.1	Trace
1	1	Trace	7	4	.2	10	Trace	Trace	Trace	Trace
—	—	—	11	11	.2	20	Trace	.01	.1	Trace
1	1	Trace	7	2	.1	0	Trace	Trace	.1	0
—	—	—	21	4	.4	0	.11	.02	.5	0
—	—	—	36	5	.4	0	.16	.02	.8	0
2	2	Trace	19	42	.7	[17]120	.08	.09	.6	Trace
1	2	1	20	96	.6	100	.07	.08	.6	Trace
—	—	—	21	11	.4	0	.01	.06	.4	0
—	1	—	8	2	.1	0	Trace	Trace	.1	0
1	4	Trace	16	13	[18].4	30	[18].05	[18].05	[18].4	Trace
—	—	—	22	147	[19].7	0	[19].12	[19].07	[19]1.0	0

[19]Iron, thiamin, riboflavin, and niacin are based on the minimum levels of enrichment specified in standards of identity promulgated under the Federal Food, Drug, and Cosmetic Act.

Food, approximate measure, and weight (in grams)		Grams	Water Per-cent	Food energy Calo-ries	Pro-tein Grams	Fat Grams
Macaroni, cooked:						
Enriched	1 cup	140	72	155	5	1
Unenriched	1 cup	140	72	155	5	1
Macaroni (enriched) and cheese, baked	1 cup	200	58	430	17	22
Muffins, with enriched white flour; muffin, 3-inch diam.	1 muffin	40	38	120	3	4
Noodles (egg noodles), cooked:						
Enriched	1 cup	160	70	200	7	2
Unenriched	1 cup	160	70	200	7	2
Oats (with or without corn) puffed, added nutrients	1 cup	25	3	100	3	1
Oatmeal or rolled oats, cooked	1 cup	240	87	130	5	2
Pancakes, 4-inch diam.:						
Plain or buttermilk (made from mix with egg and milk)	1 cake	27	51	60	2	2
Pie (piecrust made with unenriched flour):						
Sector, 4-in., $^1/_7$ of 9-in. diam. pie:						
Apple (2-crust)	1 sector	135	48	350	3	15
Cherry (2-crust)	1 sector	135	47	350	4	15
Custard (1-crust)	1 sector	130	58	285	8	14
Lemon meringue (1-crust)	1 sector	120	47	305	4	12
Mince (2-crust)	1 sector	135	43	365	3	16
Pecan (1-crust)	1 sector	118	20	490	6	27
Pumpkin (1-crust)	1 sector	130	59	275	5	15
Piecrust, baked shell for pie made with:						
Enriched flour	1 shell	180	15	900	11	60
Unenriched flour	1 shell	180	15	900	11	60
Piecrust mix including stick form:						
Package, 10-oz., for double crust	1 pkg.	284	9	1,480	20	93
Pizza (cheese) 5½-in. sector; ⅛ of 14-in. diam. pie	1 sector	75	45	185	7	6
Popcorn, popped:						
Plain, large kernel	1 cup	6	4	25	1	Trace

[19] Iron, thiamin, riboflavin, and niacin are based on the minimum levels of enrichment specified in standards of identity promulgated under the Federal Food, Drug, and Cosmetic Act.

| Fatty acids | | | Carbo-hy-drate | Cal-cium | Iron | Vita-min A value | Thia-min | Ribo-flavin | Niacin | Ascor-bic acid |
| Satu-rated (total) | Unsaturated | | | | | | | | | |
	Oleic	Lin-oleic								
Grams	*Grams*	*Grams*	*Grams*	*Milli-grams*	*Milli-grams*	*Inter-national units*	*Milli-grams*	*Milli-grams*	*Milli-grams*	*Milli-grams*
—	—	—	32	8	[19]1.3	0	[19].20	[19].11	[19]1.5	0
—	—	—	32	11	.6	0	.01	.01	.4	0
10	9	2	40	362	1.8	860	.20	.40	1.8	Trace
1	2	1	17	42	.6	40	.07	.09	.6	Trace
1	1	Trace	37	16	[19]1.4	110	[19].22	[19].13	[19]1.9	0
1	1	Trace	37	16	1.0	110	.05	.03	.6	0
—	—	—	19	44	1.2	0	0.24	0.04	0.5	0
—	—	1	23	22	1.4	0	.19	.05	.2	0
1	1	Trace	9	58	.3	70	.04	.06	.2	Trace
4	7	3	51	11	.4	40	.03	.03	.5	1
4	7	3	52	19	.4	590	.03	.03	.7	Trace
5	6	2	30	125	.8	300	.07	.21	.4	0
4	6	2	45	17	.6	200	.04	.10	.2	4
4	8	3	56	38	1.4	Trace	.09	.05	.5	1
4	16	5	60	55	3.3	190	.19	.08	.4	Trace
5	6	2	32	66	.7	3,210	.04	.13	.7	Trace
16	28	12	79	25	3.1	0	.36	.25	3.2	0
16	28	12	79	25	.9	0	.05	.05	.9	0
23	46	21	141	131	1.4	0	.11	.11	2.0	0
2	3	Trace	27	107	.7	290	.04	.12	.7	4
—	—	—	5	1	.2	—	—	.01	.1	0

Food, approximate measure, and weight (in grams)		Water	Food energy	Pro-tein	Fat
		Grams	Per-cent	Calo-ries	Grams	Grams
		Grams	*Per-cent*	*Calo-ries*	*Grams*	*Grams*
With oil and salt	1 cup	9	3	40	1	2
Sugar coated	1 cup	35	4	135	2	1
Pretzels:						
Dutch, twisted	1 pretzel	16	5	60	2	1
Thin, twisted	1 pretzel	6	5	25	1	Trace
Rice, white:						
Enriched:						
Cooked	1 cup	205	73	225	4	Trace
Instant, ready-to-serve	1 cup	165	73	180	4	Trace
Unenriched, cooked	1 cup	205	73	225	4	Trace
Parboiled, cooked	1 cup	175	73	185	4	Trace
Rice, puffed, added nutrients	1 cup	15	4	60	1	Trace
Rye wafers, whole-grain, 1⅞ by 3½ inches	2 wafers	13	6	45	2	Trace
Spaghetti, cooked, enriched	1 cup	140	72	155	5	1
Spaghetti with meat balls, and tomato sauce:						
Home recipe	1 cup	248	70	330	19	12
Canned	1 cup	250	78	260	12	10
Spaghetti in tomato sauce with cheese:						
Home recipe	1 cup	250	77	260	9	9
Canned	1 cup	250	80	190	6	2
Waffles, with enriched flour, 7-in. diam.	1 waffle	75	41	210	7	7
Waffles, made from mix, enriched, egg and milk added, 7-in. diam.	1 waffle	75	42	205	7	8
Wheat, puffed, added nutrients	1 cup	15	3	55	2	Trace
Wheat, shredded, plain	1 biscuit	25	7	90	2	1
Wheat flakes, added nutrients	1 cup	30	4	105	3	Trace
Wheat flours:						
Unsifted.	1 cup	125	12	455	13	1

[20] Iron, thiamin, and niacin are based on the minimum levels of enrichment specified in standards of identity promulgated under the Federal Food, Drug, and Cosmetic Act. Riboflavin is based on unenriched rice. When the minimum level of enrichment for riboflavin specified in the standards of identity becomes effective the value will be 0.12 milligram per cup of parboiled rice and of white rice.

| Fatty acids | | | Carbo-hy-drate | Cal-cium | Iron | Vita-min A value | Thia-min | Ribo-flavin | Niacin | Ascor-bic acid |
| Satu-rated (total) | Unsaturated | | | | | | | | | |
	Oleic	Lin-oleic								
Grams	Grams	Grams	Grams	Milli-grams	Milli-grams	Inter-national units	Milli-grams	Milli-grams	Milli-grams	Milli-grams
1	Trace	Trace	5	1	.2	—	—	.01	.2	0
—	—	—	30	2	.5	—	—	.02	.4	0
—	—	—	12	4	.2	0	Trace	Trace	.1	0
—	—	—	5	1	.1	0	Trace	Trace	Trace	0
—	—	—	50	21	[20]1.8	0	[20].23	[20].02	[20]2.1	0
—	—	—	40	5	[20]1.3	0	[20].21	[20]—	[20]1.7	0
—	—	—	50	21	.4	0	.04	.02	.8	0
—	—	—	41	33	[20]1.4	0	[20].19	[20]—	[20]2.1	0
—	—	—	13	3	.3	0	.07	.01	.7	0
—	—	—	10	7	.5	0	.04	.03	.2	0
—	—	—	32	11	[19]1.3	0	[19].20	[19].11	[19]1.5	0
4	6	1	39	124	3.7	1,590	0.25	0.30	4.0	22
2	3	4	28	53	3.3	1,000	.15	.18	2.3	5
2	5	1	37	80	2.3	1,080	.25	.18	2.3	13
1	1	1	38	40	2.8	930	.35	.28	4.5	10
2	4	1	28	85	1.3	250	.13	.19	1.0	Trace
3	3	1	27	179	1.0	170	.11	.17	.7	Trace
—	—	—	12	4	.6	0	.08	.03	1.2	0
—	—	—	20	11	.9	0	.06	.03	1.1	0
—	—	—	24	12	1.3	0	.19	.04	1.5	0
—	—	—	95	20	[19]3.6	0	[19].55	[19].33	[19]4.4	0

[19] Iron, thiamin, riboflavin, and niacin are based on the minimum levels of enrichment specified in standards of identity promulgated under the Federal Food, Drug, and Cosmetic Act.

Food, approximate measure, and weight (in grams)		Water	Food energy	Pro-tein	Fat
		Grams	*Per-cent*	*Calo-ries*	*Grams*	*Grams*

Fats, Oils

Butter:

Regular, 4 sticks per pound:

Stick	½ cup	113	16	810	1	92
Tablespoon (approx. ⅛ stick)	1 tbsp.	14	16	100	Trace	12

Whipped, 6 sticks or 2, 8-oz. containers per pound:

Stick	½ cup	76	16	540	1	61
Tablespoon (approx. ⅛ stick)	1 tbsp.	9	16	65	Trace	8

Fats, cooking:

Lard	1 cup	205	0	1,850	0	205
	1 tbsp.	13	0	115	0	13
Vegetable fats	1 cup	200	0	1,770	0	200
	1 tbsp.	13	0	110	0	13

Margarine:

Regular, 4 sticks per pound:

Stick	½ cup	113	16	815	1	92
Tablespoon (approx. ⅛ stick)	1 tbsp.	14	16	100	Trace	12

Whipped, 6 sticks per pound:

Stick	½ cup	76	16	545	1	61

Soft, 2 8-oz. tubs per pound:

Tub	1 tub	227	16	1,635	1	184
Tablespoon	1 tbsp.	14	16	100	Trace	11

Oils, salad or cooking:

Corn	1 cup	220	0	1,945	0	220
	1 tbsp.	14	0	125	0	14
Cottonseed	1 cup	220	0	1,945	0	220
	1 tbsp.	14	0	125	0	14
Olive	1 cup	220	0	1,945	0	220
	1 tbsp.	14	0	125	0	14
Peanut	1 cup	220	0	1,945	0	220
	1 tbsp.	14	0	125	0	14
Safflower	1 cup	220	0	1,945	0	220
	1 tbsp.	14	0	125	0	14

[21] Year-round average.

[22] Based on the average vitamin A content of fortified margarine. Federal specifications for fortified margarine require a minimum of 15,000 I.U. of vitamin A per pound.

| | Fatty acids | | | | | | | | | |
| | Unsaturated | | | | | | | | | |
Saturated (total)	Oleic	Linoleic	Carbohydrate	Calcium	Iron	Vitamin A value	Thiamin	Riboflavin	Niacin	Ascorbic acid
Grams	Grams	Grams	Grams	Milligrams	Milligrams	International units	Milligrams	Milligrams	Milligrams	Milligrams
51	30	3	1	23	0	[21] 3,750	—	—	—	0
6	4	Trace	Trace	3	0	[21] 470	—	—	—	0
34	20	2	Trace	15	0	[21] 2,500	—	—	—	0
4	3	Trace	Trace	2	0	[21] 310	—	—	—	0
78	94	20	0	0	0	0	0	0	0	0
5	6	1	0	0	0	0	0	0	0	0
50	100	44	0	0	0	—	0	0	0	0
3	6	3	0	0	0	—	0	0	0	0
17	46	25	1	23	0	[22] 3,750	—	—	—	0
2	6	3	Trace	3	0	[22] 470	—	—	—	0
11	31	17	Trace	15	0	[22] 2,500	—	—	—	0
34	68	68	1	45	0	[22] 7,500	—	—	—	0
2	4	4	Trace	3	0	[22] 470	—	—	—	0
22	62	117	0	0	0	—	0	0	0	0
1	4	7	0	0	0	—	0	0	0	0
55	46	110	0	0	0	—	0	0	0	0
4	3	7	0	0	0	—	0	0	0	0
24	167	15	0	0	0	—	0	0	0	0
2	11	1	0	0	0	—	0	0	0	0
40	103	64	0	0	0	—	0	0	0	0
3	7	4	0	0	0	—	0	0	0	0
18	37	165	0	0	0	—	0	0	0	0
1	2	10	0	0	0	—	0	0	0	0

Food, approximate measure, and weight (in grams)		Water	Food energy	Pro-tein	Fat
		Grams	*Per-cent*	*Calo-ries*	*Grams* *Grams*
Soybean	1 cup	220	0	1,945	0	220
	1 tbsp.	14	0	125	0	14
Salad dressings:						
Blue cheese	1 tbsp.	15	32	75	1	8
Commercial, mayonnaise type:						
Regular	1 tbsp.	15	41	65	Trace	6
Special dietary, low-calorie	1 tbsp.	16	81	20	Trace	2
French:						
Regular	1 tbsp.	16	39	65	Trace	6
Special dietary, low-fat with artificial sweeteners	1 tbsp.	15	95	Trace	Trace	Trace
Mayonnaise	1 tbsp.	14	15	100	Trace	11
Thousand island	1 tbsp.	16	32	80	Trace	8
Sugars, Sweets						
Cake icings:						
Chocolate made with milk and table fat	1 cup	275	14	1,035	0	38
Coconut (with boiled icing)	1 cup	166	15	605	3	13
Creamy fudge from mix with water only	1 cup	245	15	830	7	16
White, boiled	1 cup	94	18	300	1	0
Candy:						
Caramels, plain or chocolate	1 oz.	28	8	115	1	3
Chocolate, milk, plain	1 oz.	28	1	145	2	9
Chocolate-coated peanuts	1 oz.	28	1	160	5	12
Fudge, plain	1 oz.	28	8	115	1	4
Hard	1 oz.	28	1	110	0	Trace
Marshmallows	1 oz.	28	17	90	1	Trace
Chocolate-flavored sirup or topping:						
Fudge type	1 fl. oz.	38	25	125	2	5
Chocolate-flavored beverage powder (approx. 4 heaping teaspoons per oz.):						
With nonfat dry milk	1 oz.	28	2	100	5	1
Honey, strained or extracted	1 tbsp.	21	17	65	Trace	0
Jams and preserves	1 tbsp.	20	29	55	Trace	Trace
Jellies	1 tbsp.	18	29	50	Trace	Trace

Fatty acids										
Saturated (total)	Unsaturated		Carbohydrate	Calcium	Iron	Vitamin A value	Thiamin	Riboflavin	Niacin	Ascorbic acid
	Oleic	Linoleic								
Grams	Grams	Grams	Grams	Milligrams	Milligrams	International units	Milligrams	Milligrams	Milligrams	Milligrams
33	44	114	0	0	0	—	0	0	0	0
2	3	7	0	0	0	—	0	0	0	0
2	2	4	1	12	Trace	30	Trace	0.02	Trace	Trace
1	1	3	2	2	Trace	30	Trace	Trace	Trace	—
Trace	Trace	1	1	3	Trace	40	Trace	Trace	Trace	—
1	1	3	3	2	.1	—	—	—	—	—
—	—	—	Trace	2	.1	—	—	—	—	—
2	2	6	Trace	3	.1	40	Trace	.01	Trace	—
1	2	4	3	2	.1	50	Trace	Trace	Trace	Trace
21	11	1	185	165	3.3	580	.06	.28	.6	1
11	1	Trace	124	10	.8	0	.02	.07	.3	0
5	8	3	183	96	2.7	Trace	.05	.20	.7	Trace
—	—	—	76	2	Trace	0	Trace	.03	Trace	0
2	1	Trace	22	42	.4	Trace	.01	.05	.1	Trace
5	3	Trace	16	65	.3	80	.02	.10	.1	Trace
3	6	2	11	33	.4	Trace	.10	.05	2.1	Trace
2	1	Trace	21	22	.3	Trace	.01	.03	.1	Trace
—	—	—	28	6	.5	0	0	0	0	0
—	—	—	23	5	.5	0	0	Trace	Trace	0
3	2	Trace	20	48	.5	60	.02	.08	.2	Trace
Trace	Trace	Trace	20	167	.5	10	.04	.21	.2	1
—	—	—	17	1	.1	0	Trace	.01	.1	Trace
—	—	—	14	4	.2	Trace	Trace	.01	Trace	Trace
—	—	—	13	4	.3	Trace	Trace	.01	Trace	1

Food, approximate measure, and weight (in grams)		Grams	Water Per-cent	Food energy Calo-ries	Pro-tein Grams	Fat Grams
Molasses, cane:						
Light (first extraction)	1 tbsp.	20	24	50	—	—
Blackstrap (third extraction)	1 tbsp.	20	24	45	—	—
Sirups:						
Table blends, chiefly corn, light and dark	1 tbsp.	21	24	60	0	0
Sugars:						
Brown, firm packed	1 cup	220	2	820	0	0
White:						
Granulated	1 cup	200	Trace	770	0	0
	1 tbsp.	11	Trace	40	0	0
Powdered, stirred before measuring	1 cup	120	Trace	460	0	0
Miscellaneous Items						
Barbecue sauce	1 cup	250	81	230	4	17
Beverages, alcoholic:						
Beer	12 fl. oz.	360	92	150	1	0
Gin, rum, vodka, whiskey:						
80-proof	1½ fl. oz. jigger	42	67	100	—	—
86-proof	1½ fl. oz. jigger	42	64	105	—	—
90-proof	1½ fl. oz. jigger	42	62	110	—	—
94-proof	1½ fl. oz. jigger	42	60	115	—	—
100-proof	1½ fl. oz. jigger	42	58	125	—	—
Wines:						
Dessert	3½ fl. oz. glass	103	77	140	Trace	0
Table	3½ fl. oz. glass	102	86	85	Trace	0
Beverages, carbonated, sweetened, nonalcoholic:						
Carbonated water	12 fl. oz.	366	92	115	0	0
Cola type	12 fl. oz.	369	90	145	0	0

Fatty acids										
Saturated (total)	Unsaturated		Carbohydrate	Calcium	Iron	Vitamin A value	Thiamin	Riboflavin	Niacin	Ascorbic acid
	Oleic	Linoleic								
Grams	Grams	Grams	Grams	Milligrams	Milligrams	International units	Milligrams	Milligrams	Milligrams	Milligrams
—	—	—	13	33	.9	—	.01	.01	Trace	—
—	—	—	11	137	3.2	—	.02	.04	.4	—
—	—	—	15	9	.8	0	0	0	0	0
—	—	—	212	187	7.5	0	.02	.07	.4	0
—	—	—	199	0	.2	0	0	0	0	0
—	—	—	11	0	Trace	0	0	0	0	0
—	—	—	119	0	.1	0	0	0	0	0
2	5	9	20	53	2.0	900	.03	.03	.8	13
—	—	—	14	18	Trace	—	.01	.11	2.2	—
—	—	—	Trace	—	—	—	—	—	—	—
—	—	—	Trace	—	—	—	—	—	—	—
—	—	—	Trace	—	—	—	—	—	—	—
—	—	—	Trace	—	—	—	—	—	—	—
—	—	—	Trace	—	—	—	—	—	—	—
—	—	—	8	8	—	—	.01	.02	.2	—
—	—	—	4	9	.4	—	Trace	.01	.1	—
—	—	—	29	—	—	0	0	0	0	0
—	—	—	37	—	—	0	0	0	0	0

Food, approximate measure, and weight (in grams)		Grams	Water Per-cent	Food energy Calo-ries	Pro-tein Grams	Fat Grams
Fruit-flavored sodas and Tom Collins mixes	12 fl. oz.	372	88	170	0	0
Ginger ale	12 fl. oz.	366	92	115	0	0
Root beer	12 fl. oz.	370	90	150	0	0
Bouillon cubes, approx. ½ in.	1 cube	4	4	5	1	Trace
Chocolate:						
Bitter or baking	1 oz.	28	2	145	3	15
Semi-sweet, small pieces	1 cup	170	1	860	7	61
Gelatin	1 envelope	7	13	25	6	Trace
Gelatin dessert, prepared with water	1 cup	240	84	140	4	0
Popcorn. See Grain Products.						
Popsicle, 3 fl. oz. size	1 popsicle	95	80	70	0	0
Pudding, home recipe with starch base:						
Chocolate	1 cup	260	66	385	8	12
Vanilla (blanc mange)	1 cup	255	76	285	9	10
Pudding mix, dry form, 4-oz. package	1 pkg.	113	2	410	3	2
Sherbet	1 cup	193	67	260	2	2
Soups:						
Canned, condensed, ready-to-serve:						
Prepared with an equal volume of milk:						
Cream of chicken	1 cup	245	85	180	7	10
Cream of mushroom	1 cup	245	83	215	7	14
Tomato	1 cup	250	84	175	7	7
Prepared with an equal volume of water:						
Bean with pork	1 cup	250	84	170	8	6
Beef broth, bouillon consomme	1 cup	240	96	30	5	0
Beef noodle	1 cup	240	93	70	4	3
Clam chowder, Manhattan type (with tomatoes, without milk)	1 cup	245	92	80	2	3
Cream of chicken	1 cup	240	92	95	3	6
Cream of mushroom	1 cup	240	90	135	2	10
Minestrone	1 cup	245	90	105	5	3
Split pea	1 cup	245	85	145	9	3

Fatty acids										
Saturated (total)	Unsaturated		Carbo-hy-drate	Cal-cium	Iron	Vita-min A value	Thia-min	Ribo-flavin	Niacin	Ascor-bic acid
	Oleic	Lin-oleic								
Grams	Grams	Grams	Grams	Milli-grams	Milli-grams	Inter-national units	Milli-grams	Milli-grams	Milli-grams	Milli-grams
—	—	—	45	—	—	0	0	0	0	0
—	—	—	29	—	—	0	0	0	0	0
—	—	—	39	—	—	0	0	0	0	0
—	—	—	Trace	—	—	—	—	—	—	—
8	6	Trace	8	22	1.9	20	.01	.07	.4	0
34	22	1	97	51	4.4	30	.02	.14	.9	0
—	—	—	0	—	—	—	—	—	—	
—	—	—	34	—	—	—	—	—	—	—
0	0	0	18	0	Trace	0	0	0	0	0
7	4	Trace	67	250	1.3	390	.05	.36	.3	1
5	3	Trace	41	298	Trace	410	.08	.41	.3	2
1	1	Trace	103	23	1.8	Trace	.02	.08	.5	0
—	—	—	59	31	Trace	120	.02	.06	Trace	4
3	3	3	15	172	.5	610	.05	.27	.7	2
4	4	5	16	191	.5	250	.05	.34	.7	1
3	2	1	23	168	.8	1,200	.10	.25	1.3	15
1	2	2	22	63	2.3	650	.13	.08	1.0	3
—	—	—	3	Trace	.5	Trace	Trace	.02	1.2	—
1	1	1	7	7	1.0	50	.05	.07	1.0	Trace
—	—	—	12	34	1.0	880	.02	.02	1.0	—
1	2	3	8	24	.5	410	.02	.05	.5	Trace
1	3	5	10	41	.5	70	.02	.12	.7	Trace
—	—	—	14	37	1.0	2,350	.07	.05	1.0	—
1	2	Trace	21	29	1.5	440	0.25	0.15	1.5	1

Food, approximate measure, and weight (in grams)		Water	Food energy	Pro-tein	Fat
		Grams	*Per-cent*	*Calo-ries*	*Grams* *Grams*
Tomato	1 cup	245	90	90	2	3
Vegetable beef	1 cup	245	92	80	5	2
Vegetarian	1 cup	245	92	80	2	2
Dehydrated, dry form:						
Chicken noodle (2-oz. package)	1 pkg.	57	6	220	8	6
Onion mix (1½-oz. package)	1 pkg.	43	3	150	6	5
Tomato vegetable with noodles (2½-oz. pkg.)	1 pkg.	71	4	245	6	6
Tapioca desserts:						
Apple	1 cup	250	70	295	1	Trace
Cream pudding	1 cup	165	72	220	8	8
Tartar sauce	1 tbsp.	14	34	75	Trace	8
Vinegar	1 tbsp.	15	94	Trace	Trace	0
White sauce, medium	1 cup	250	73	405	10	31

Fatty acids										
Saturated (total)	Unsaturated		Carbo-hy-drate	Cal-cium	Iron	Vita-min A value	Thia-min	Ribo-flavin	Niacin	Ascor-bic acid
	Oleic	Lin-oleic								
Grams	Grams	Grams	Grams	Milli-grams	Milli-grams	Inter-national units	Milli-grams	Milli-grams	Milli-grams	Milli-grams
Trace	1	1	16	15	.7	1,000	.05	.05	1.2	12
—	—	—	10	12	.7	2,700	.05	.05	1.0	—
—	—	—	13	20	1.0	2,940	.05	.05	1.0	—
2	3	1	33	34	1.4	190	.30	.15	2.4	3
1	2	1	23	42	.6	30	.05	.03	.3	6
2	3	1	45	33	1.4	1,700	.21	.13	1.8	18
—	—	—	74	8	.5	30	Trace	Trace	Trace	Trace
4	3	Trace	28	173	.7	480	.07	.30	.2	.2
1	1	4	1	3	.1	30	Trace	Trace	Trace	Trace
—	—	—	1	1	.1	—	—	—	—	—
19	8	1	22	288	.5	1,150	.10	.43	.5	2

APPENDIX 2

Nutrition and Your Health: Dietary Guidelines for Americans*

- Eat a variety of foods
- Maintain ideal weight
- Avoid too much fat, saturated fat, and cholesterol
- Eat foods with adequate starch and fiber
- Avoid too much sugar
- Avoid too much sodium
- If you drink alcohol, do so in moderation

Eat a Variety of Foods

You need about forty different nutrients to stay healthy. These include vitamins and minerals, as well as amino acids (from proteins), essential fatty acids (from vegetable oils and animal fats), and sources of energy (calories from carbohydrates, proteins, and fats). These nutrients are in the foods you normally eat.

Most foods contain more than one nutrient. Milk, for example, provides proteins, fats, sugars, riboflavin and other B-vitamins, vitamin A, calcium, and phosphorus — among other nutrients.

No single food item supplies all the essential nutrients in the amounts that you need. Milk, for instance, contains very little iron or vitamin C. You should, therefore, eat a variety of foods to assure an adequate diet.

The greater the variety, the less likely you are to develop either a deficiency or an excess of any single nutrient. Variety also reduces your likelihood of being exposed to excessive amounts of contaminants in any single food item.

One way to assure variety and, with it, a well-balanced diet is to

*These dietary guidelines were issued in 1980 by the U.S. Department of Agriculture and the U.S. Department of Health, Education, and Welfare.

select foods each day from each of several major groups: for example, fruits and vegetables; cereals, breads, and grains; meats, poultry, eggs, and fish; dry peas and beans, such as soybeans, kidney beans, lima beans, and black-eyed peas, which are good vegetable sources of protein; and milk, cheese, and yogurt.

Fruits and vegetables are excellent sources of vitamins, especially vitamins C and A. Whole grain and enriched breads, cereals, and grain products provide B-vitamins, iron, and energy. Meats supply protein, fat, iron and other minerals, as well as several vitamins, including thiamine and vitamin B_{12}. Dairy products are major sources of calcium and other nutrients.

To Assure Yourself an Adequate Diet

Eat a variety of foods daily, including selections of
- Fruits
- Vegetables
- Whole grain and enriched breads, cereals, and grain products
- Milk, cheese, and yogurt
- Meats, poultry, fish, eggs
- Legumes (dry peas and beans)

There are no known advantages to consuming excess amounts of any nutrient. You will rarely need to take vitamin or mineral supplements if you eat a wide variety of foods. There are a few important exceptions to this general statement:

• *Women in their childbearing years* may need to take iron supplements to replace the iron they lose with menstrual bleeding. Women who are no longer menstruating should not take iron supplements routinely.

• *Women who are pregnant or who are breastfeeding* need more of many nutrients, especially iron, folic acid, vitamin A, calcium, and sources of energy (calories from carbohydrates, proteins, and fats). Detailed advice should come from their physicians or from dietitians.

• *Elderly or very inactive people* may eat relatively little food. Thus, they should pay special attention to avoiding foods that are high in calories but low in other essential nutrients — for example, fat, oils, alcohol, and sugars.

Infants also have special nutritional needs. Healthy full-term infants should be breastfed unless there are special problems. The nutrients in human breast milk tend to be digested and absorbed more easily than those in cow's milk. In addition, breast milk may serve to transfer immunity to some diseases from the mother to the infant.

Normally, most babies do not need solid foods until they are 3 to 6 months old. At that time, other foods can be introduced gradually. Prolonged breast or bottlefeeding — without solid foods or supplemental iron — can result in iron deficiency.

You should not add salt or sugar to the baby's foods. Infants do not need these "encouragements" — if they are really hungry. The foods themselves contain enough salt and sugar; extra is not necessary.

To Assure Your Baby an Adequate Diet

- Breastfeed unless there are special problems
- Delay other foods until baby is 3 to 6 months old
- Do not add salt or sugar to baby's food

Maintain Ideal Weight

If you are too fat, your chances of developing some chronic disorders are increased. Obesity is associated with high blood pressure, increased levels of blood fats (triglycerides) and cholesterol, and the most common type of diabetes. All of these, in turn, are associated with increased risks of heart attacks and strokes. Thus, you should try to maintain "ideal" weight.

But, how do you determine what the ideal weight is for you?

There is no absolute answer. The table on the following page shows "acceptable" ranges for most adults. If you have been obese since childhood, you may find it difficult to reach or to maintain your weight within the acceptable range. For most people, their weight should not be more than it was when they were young adults (20 or 25 years old).

It is not well understood why some people can eat much more than others and still maintain normal weight. However, one thing

---

To Improve Eating Habits

- Eat slowly
- Prepare smaller portions
- Avoid "seconds"

is definite: to lose weight, you must take in fewer calories than you burn. This means that you must either select foods containing fewer calories or you must increase your activity — or both.

If you need to lose weight, do so gradually. Steady loss of 1 to 2 pounds a week — until you reach your goal — is relatively safe and more likely to be maintained. Long-term success depends upon acquiring new and better habits of eating and exercise. That is perhaps why "crash" diets usually fail in the long run.

Do not try to lose weight too rapidly. Avoid crash diets that are severely restricted in the variety of foods they allow. Diets containing fewer than 800 calories may be hazardous. Some people have developed kidney stones, disturbing psychological changes, and other complications while following such diets. A few people have died suddenly and without warning.

Gradual increase of everyday physical activities like walking or climbing stairs can be very helpful. The chart on page 307 gives the calories used per hour in different activities.

A pound of body fat contains 3500 calories. To lose 1 pound of fat,

Suggested Body Weights

Range of Acceptable Weight

Height (feet-inches)	Men (Pounds)	Women (Pounds)
4'10"		92–119
4'11"		94–122
5'0"		96–125
5'1"		99–128
5'2"	112–141	102–131
5'3"	115–144	105–134
5'4"	118–148	108–138
5'5"	121–152	111–142
5'6"	124–156	114–146
5'7"	128–161	118–150
5'8"	132–166	122–154
5'9"	136–170	126–158
5'10"	140–174	130–163
5'11"	144–179	134–168
6'0"	148–184	138–173
6'1"	152–189	
6'2"	156–194	
6'3"	160–199	
6'4"	164–204	

NOTE: Height without shoes; weight without clothes.
SOURCE: HEW conference on obesity, 1973.

Approximate Energy Expenditure by a 150 Pound Person in Various Activities

Activity	Calories per hour
Lying down or sleeping	80
Sitting	100
Driving an automobile	120
Standing	140
Domestic work	180
Walking, 2½ mph	210
Bicycling, 5½ mph	210
Gardening	220
Golf; lawn mowing, power mower	250
Bowling	270
Walking, 3¾ mph	300
Swimming, ¼ mph	300
Square dancing, volleyball; roller skating	350
Wood chopping or sawing	400
Tennis	420
Skiing, 10 mph	600
Squash and handball	600
Bicycling, 13 mph	660
Running, 10 mph	900

SOURCE: Based on material prepared by Robert E. Johnson, M.D., Ph.D., and colleagues, University of Illinois.

To Lose Weight

- Increase physical activity
- Eat less fat and fatty foods
- Eat less sugar and sweets
- Avoid too much alcohol

---

you will need to burn 3500 calories more than you consume. If you burn 500 calories more a day than you consume, you will lose 1 pound of fat a week. Thus, if you normally burn 1700 calories a day, you can theoretically expect to lose a pound of fat each week if you adhere to a 1200-calorie-per-day diet.

Do not attempt to reduce your weight below the acceptable

range. Severe weight loss may be associated with nutrient deficiencies, menstrual irregularities, infertility, hair loss, skin changes, cold intolerance, severe constipation, psychiatric disturbances, and other complications.

If you lose weight suddenly or for unknown reasons, see a physician. Unexplained weight loss may be an early clue to an unsuspected underlying disorder.

Avoid Too Much Fat, Saturated Fat, and Cholesterol

If you have a high blood cholesterol level, you have a greater chance of having a heart attack. Other factors can also increase your risk of heart attack — high blood pressure and cigarette smoking, for example — but high blood cholesterol is clearly a major dietary risk indicator.

Populations like ours with diets high in saturated fats and cholesterol tend to have high blood cholesterol levels. Individuals within these populations usually have greater risks of having heart attacks than people eating low-fat, low-cholesterol diets.

Eating extra saturated fat and cholesterol will increase blood cholesterol levels in most people. However, there are wide variations among people — related to heredity and the way each person's body uses cholesterol.

Some people can consume diets high in saturated fats and cholesterol and still keep normal blood cholesterol levels. Other people, unfortunately, have high blood cholesterol levels even if they eat low-fat, low-cholesterol diets.

There is controversy about what recommendations are appropriate for healthy Americans. But for the U.S. population *as a whole*,

---

To Avoid Too Much Fat, Saturated Fat, and Cholesterol

- Choose lean meat, fish, poultry, dry beans and peas as your protein sources
- Moderate your use of eggs and organ meats (such as liver)
- Limit your intake of butter, cream, hydrogenated margarines, shortenings and coconut oil, and foods made from such products
- Trim excess fat off meats
- Broil, bake, or boil rather than fry
- Read labels carefully to determine both amount and types of fat contained in foods

---

reduction in our current intake of total fat, saturated fat, and cholesterol is sensible. This suggestion is especially appropriate for people who have high blood pressure or who smoke.

The recommendations are not meant to prohibit the use of any specific food item or to prevent you from eating a variety of foods. For example, eggs and organ meats (such as liver) contain cholesterol, but they also contain many essential vitamins and minerals, as well as protein. Such items can be eaten in moderation, as long as your overall cholesterol intake is not excessive. If you prefer whole milk to skim milk, you can reduce your intake of fats from foods other than milk.

Eat Foods with Adequate Starch and Fiber

The major sources of energy in the average U.S. diet are carbohydrates and fats. (Proteins and alcohol also supply energy, but to a lesser extent.) If you limit your fat intake, you should increase your calories from carbohydrates to supply your body's energy needs.

In trying to reduce your weight to "ideal" levels, carbohydrates have an advantage over fats: carbohydrates contain less than half the number of calories per ounce than fats.

Complex carbohydrate foods are better than *simple* carbohydrates in this regard. Simple carbohydrates — such as sugars — provide calories but little else in the way of nutrients. Complex carbohydrate foods — such as beans, peas, nuts, seeds, fruits and vegetables, and whole grain breads, cereals, and products — contain many essential nutrients in addition to calories.

Increasing your consumption of certain complex carbohydrates can also help increase dietary fiber. The average American diet is relatively low in fiber. Eating more foods high in fiber tends to reduce the symptoms of chronic constipation, diverticulosis, and some types of "irritable bowel." There is also concern that low fiber diets might increase the risk of developing cancer of the colon, but whether this is true is not yet known.

To make sure you get enough fiber in your diet, you should eat fruits and vegetables, whole grain breads and cereals. There is no reason to add fiber to foods that do not already contain it.

To Eat More Complex Carbohydrates Daily

- Substitute starches for fats and sugars
- Select foods which are good sources of fiber and starch, such as whole grain breads and cereals, fruits and vegetables, beans, peas, and nuts

Avoid Too Much Sugar

The major health hazard from eating too much sugar is tooth decay (dental caries). The risk of caries is not simply a matter of how much sugar you eat. The risk increases the more frequently you eat sugar and sweets, especially if you eat between meals, and if you eat foods that stick to the teeth. For example, frequent snacks of sticky candy, or dates, or daylong use of soft drinks may be more harmful than adding sugar to your morning cup of coffee — at least as far as your teeth are concerned.

Obviously, there is more to healthy teeth than avoiding sugars. Careful dental hygiene and exposure to adequate amounts of fluoride in the water are especially important.

Contrary to widespread opinion, too much sugar in your diet does not seem to cause diabetes. The most common type of diabetes is seen in obese adults, and avoiding sugar, without correcting the overweight, will not solve the problem. There is also no convincing evidence that sugar causes heart attacks or blood vessel diseases.

Estimates indicate that Americans use on the average more than 130 pounds of sugars and sweeteners a year. This means the risk of tooth decay is increased not only by the sugar in the sugar bowl but by the sugars and syrups in jams, jellies, candies, cookies, soft drinks, cakes, and pies, as well as sugars found in products such as breakfast cereals, catsup, flavored milks, and ice cream. Frequently, the ingredient label will provide a clue to the amount of sugars in a product.

To Avoid Excessive Sugars

- Use less of all sugars, including white sugar, brown sugar, raw sugar, honey, and syrups
- Eat less of foods containing these sugars, such as candy, soft drinks, ice cream, cakes, cookies
- Select fresh fruits or fruits canned without sugar or light syrup rather than heavy syrup
- Read food labels for clues on sugar content — if the names sucrose, glucose, maltose, dextrose, lactose, fructose, or syrups appear first, then there is a large amount of sugar
- Remember, how often you eat sugar is as important as how much sugar you eat

Avoid Too Much Sodium

Table salt contains sodium and chloride — both are essential elements.

Sodium is also present in many beverages and foods that we eat, especially in certain processed foods, condiments, sauces, pickled foods, salty snacks, and sandwich meats. Baking soda, baking powder, monosodium glutamate (MSG), soft drinks, and even many medications (many antacids, for instance) contain sodium.

It is not surprising that adults in the United States take in much more sodium than they need.

The major hazard of excessive sodium is for persons who have high blood pressure. Not everyone is equally susceptible. In the United States, approximately 17 percent of adults have high blood pressure. Sodium intake is but one of the factors known to affect blood pressure. Obesity, in particular, seems to play a major role.

In populations with low-sodium intakes, high blood pressure is rare. In contrast, in populations with high-sodium intakes, high blood pressure is common. If people with high blood pressure severely restrict their sodium intakes, their blood pressures will *usually* fall — although not always to normal levels.

At present, there is no good way to predict who will develop high blood pressure, though certain groups, such as blacks, have a higher incidence. Low-sodium diets might help some of these people avoid high blood pressure if they could be identified before they develop the condition.

Since most Americans eat more sodium than is needed, consider reducing your sodium intake. Use less table salt. Eat sparingly those foods to which large amounts of sodium have been added.

To Avoid Too Much Sodium

- Learn to enjoy the unsalted flavors of foods
- Cook with only small amounts of added salt
- Add little or no salt to food at the table
- Limit your intake of salty foods, such as potato chips, pretzels, salted nuts and popcorn, condiments (soy sauce, steak sauce, garlic salt), cheese, pickled foods, cured meats
- Read food labels carefully to determine the amounts of sodium in processed foods and snack items

Remember that up to half of sodium intake may be "hidden," either as part of the naturally occurring food or, more often, as part of a preservative or flavoring agent that has been added.

If You Drink Alcohol, Do So in Moderation

Alcoholic beverages tend to be high in calories and low in other nutrients. Even moderate drinkers may need to drink less if they wish to achieve ideal weight.

On the other hand, heavy drinkers may lose their appetites for foods containing essential nutrients. Vitamin and mineral deficiencies occur commonly in heavy drinkers — in part, because of poor intake, but also because alcohol alters the absorption and use of some essential nutrients.

Sustained or excessive alcohol consumption by pregnant women has caused birth defects. Pregnant women should limit alcohol intake to 2 ounces or less on any single day.

Heavy drinking may also cause a variety of serious conditions, such as cirrhosis of the liver and some neurological disorders. Cancer of the throat and neck is much more common in people who drink and smoke than in people who don't.

One or two drinks daily appear to cause no harm in adults. If you drink you should do so in moderation.

• Remember, if you drink alcohol, do so in moderation

General Index
Index of Recipes

General Index

Index of Recipes